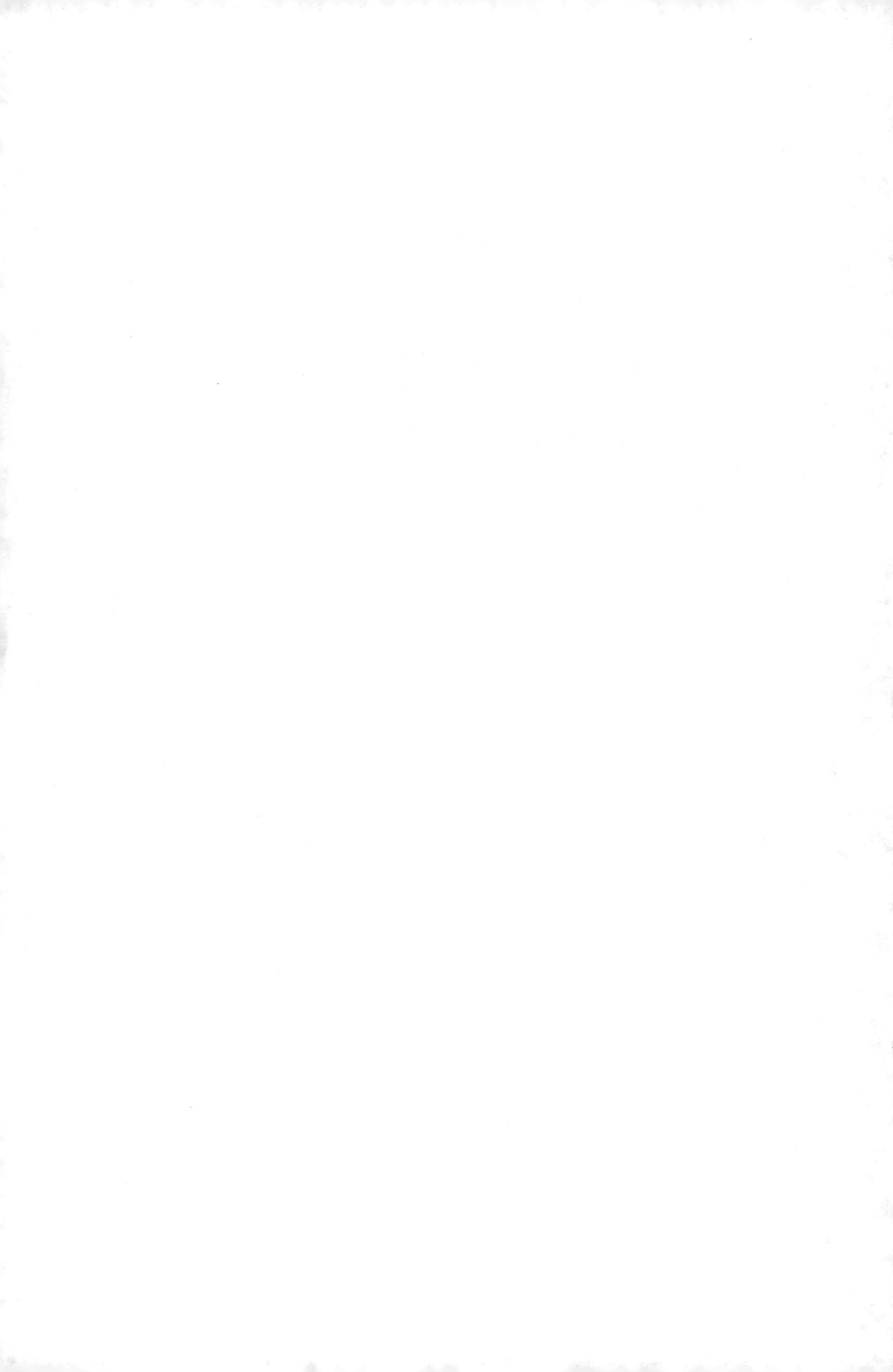

God Said Not Yet!

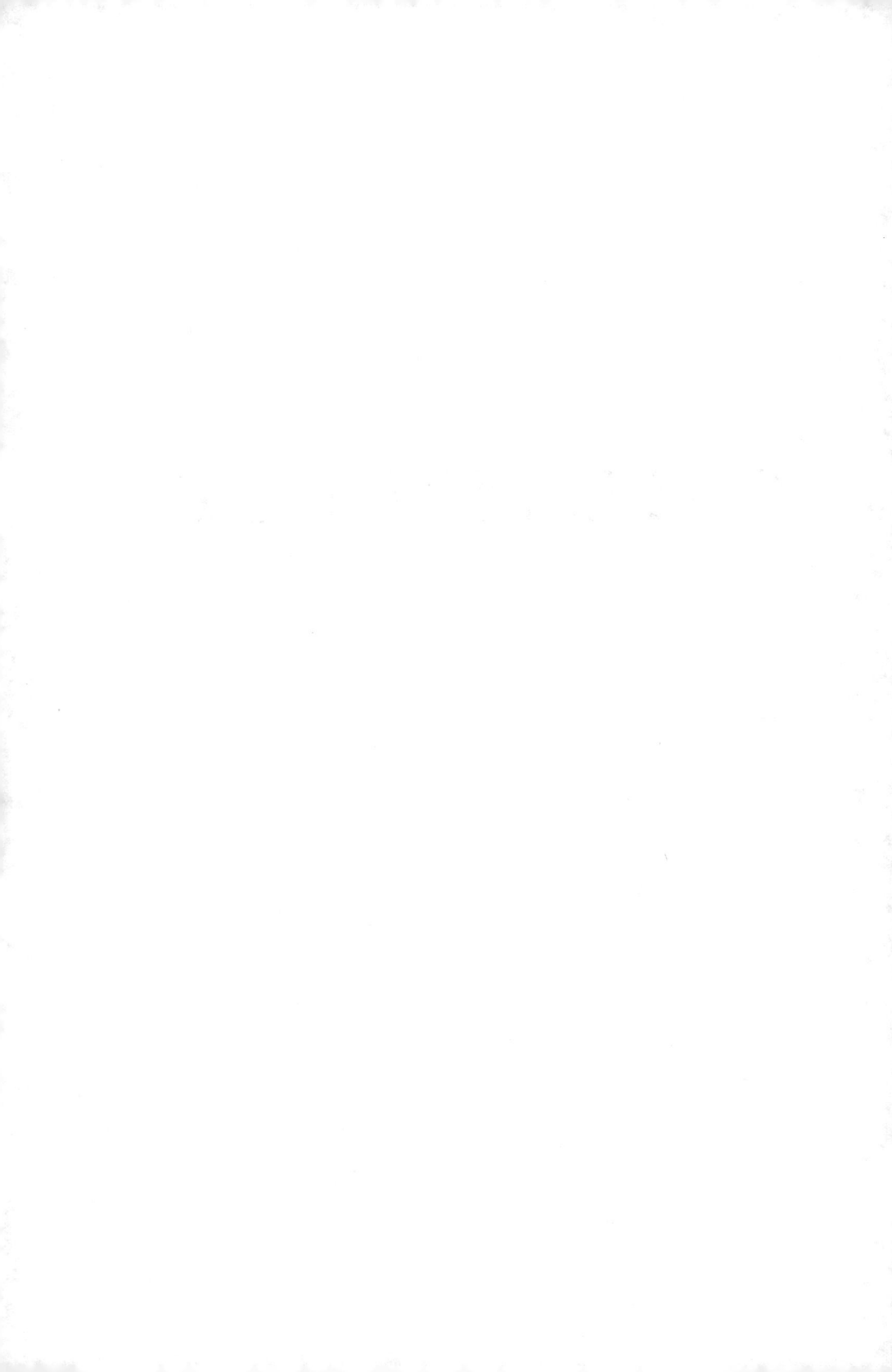

God Said, Not Yet!

One Man's Experience With "Terminal" Cancer

by

Daniel Edward Neff

This book is a personal account of Daniel's experience with cancer. All statements and assertions in this book are solely personal opinions (unless otherwise footnoted) and are not meant to be construed as professional advice or information.

Publisher: Daniel Edward Neff

57 Half Timber Drive

Marion, NC 28752

ISBN: 1451562306

EAN-13:   9781451562309

Cover Design: Daniel Edward Neff

Photography: Daniel Edward Neff

Book Design: Daniel Edward Neff

Printed in the United States by CreateSpace

Bulk Purchases contact: neffmoorebooks@yahoo.com

Table of Contents

Foreword

This is a book I have wanted to write since I first realized I was going to recover from "terminal" cancer in 2001. Over the years, since recovering from "terminal" cancer, I have shared my story with countless people, recounting God's miracles and the leap of faith I had to take (walking away from medical treatment when it looked certain I was going to die). Many people would remark, "You should write a book." I knew that there was so much to my story that it needed to be told to more people than I could reach alone.

As soon as I started recovering and feeling better, I knew that I was supposed to jump back into youth work. Between moving, trying to start a home for kids in Ohio, then moving to Maine and working in a group home, I never had the time or the energy to write this story. Working with teenagers in a group home is a lot more exhausting than it seems. Most people think that being a houseparent is all about cooking meals, watching movies or playing games, then filling out paperwork. But there is a lot more to it than that: whether it is the stress of dealing with a defiant teenager, or experiencing heartache when hearing about all the abuse and neglect a kid went through, the emotional exhaustion you experience can be very draining. Therefore, whenever we had time off, we traveled or rested or engaged in recreation to recharge our batteries.

We left Maine, thinking we were done working with youth in a residential setting. After a two year break in Kentucky, however, it was clear that we were called to get back into this work one last time. We found a place in Western North Carolina, interviewed for the job, and accepted the offer to be houseparents. We packed up our belongings and headed to the Tar Heel State.

After we settled in to our group home in North Carolina, I started making more of an effort to go ahead and start on the book about my experience with cancer. I didn't make tremendous progress, but it was a start. When the administration defenestrated us in the fall of 2009, we were shocked and slandered, but it turned out to be a blessing in disguise. I suddenly had, through no plan of my own, plenty of time on my hands. I set out to finally write this book.

We can't always see the end of the path (okay we never can), but if we trust God, He will illuminate the next couple of steps. All we have to do is rely on Him and know that He works all things together for good for those that love Him. Rather than sit around and feel sorry for myself (okay I did a little bit of that....Linda, I don't need your comments here), I worked hard on my book, researched the publishing process, and got involved in a Toastmasters Club (knowing that at some point I would need to get out and promote my book). Toastmasters International is a non-profit educational organization that teaches public speaking and leadership skills through a worldwide network of meeting locations. I already had some experience in public speaking, and it doesn't terrify me, but I knew that I could use refining and development of my skills. The book and the story would sell the book, but the quality of the presentation would dictate how much it would sell. I joined Toastmasters to equip myself to promote my book; I had no idea how much I would enjoy the camaraderie and how much it would improve my communication skills.

I decided on the self-publishing route, after hitting a few obstacles in the traditional route (finding an agent, finding a publisher willing to take on the project, etc.). In the end, I think the self-publishing route is probably best for my story. My experience with cancer and facing death is saturated with my Christian faith, and I am afraid that a publishing house would have wanted to water that down significantly. Without God's provision and guidance, and the gift of faith to step out in the face of death, there is nothing to my story. I am not ashamed of my faith or my Savior Jesus Christ, and I am free to tell this story of my experience with "terminal" cancer uncensored.

Acknowledgments

I would like to thank God for: bringing me through cancer; giving me the faith to trust Him in the face of death; providing for all our needs; and making this book possible. God's peace, the peace that transcends all understanding, was instrumental in freeing me from fear and enabling me to walk away from medical treatment.

I am grateful to my lovely wife Linda who was a rock of support during my illness and a tremendous help to me in writing this book. My son Daniel, who is the apple of my eye, was a source of inspiration when I was sick, and helped design the book cover.

Dusty, our Golden Retriever who passed away in 2008 at the age of 14 (98 to you and me), was a wonderful dog, and a warm, fuzzy companion to all of us when I was sick. Johnny, our new Golden Retriever, born in January 2009, is a constant source of fun, joy, consternation and challenge, because he is a spoiled horse puppy.

I would like to thank St. Vincent's Catholic Hospital in Jacksonville, FL. I am grateful to all the caring nurses (and the rest of the medical staff) at St. Vincent's who took me in and treated me when I was sick.

I am eternally grateful for all the people who prayed for me while I was battling cancer. Through friends and family, there were churches all over America praying for me. Although too numerous to list here, we are eternally grateful to the church families of family and friends who prayed for us and helped us in many ways during our time of need. Thanks to the Bengals' fan internet forum, there were people all over the world praying for me (yes there are Bengals' fans in other countries, believe it or not).

Linda and I are eternally grateful to all of our family and friends, and our family at St. Peter's Episcopal Church in Jacksonville, FL (where we attended while we lived there), who were so supportive during my time of illness. Your emotional support, prayers, and financial assistance can never be repaid.

I would also like to thank all the members of our church family at St. Paul's Episcopal Church in Lake James, North Carolina, who were very generous and helpful during a difficult time of unemployment.

To avoid leaving anyone out, I will refrain from naming all the individuals who provided for our many needs and prayed for us during my battle with cancer. We truly appreciate all of our family and friends.

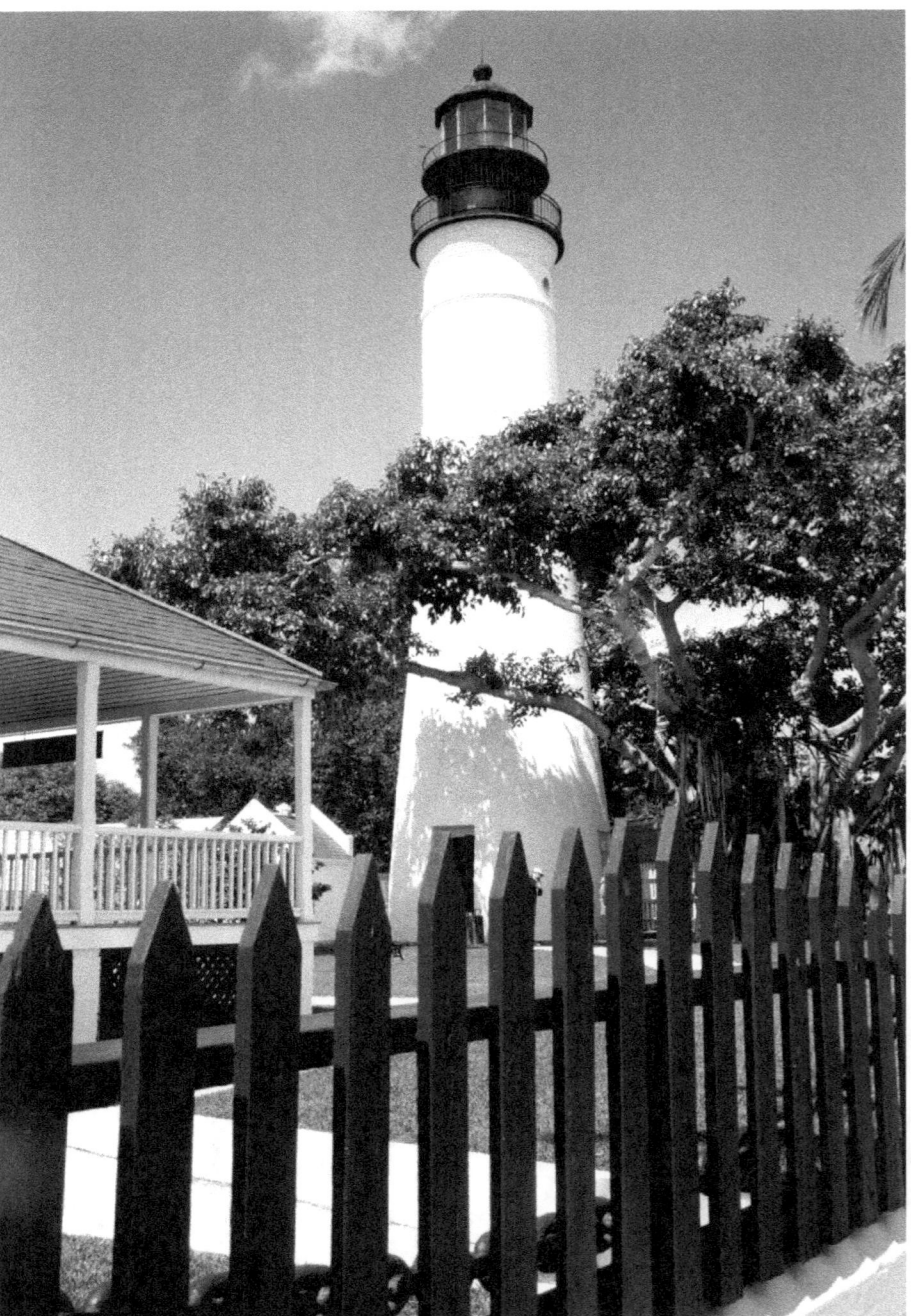

Chapter 1

He Stopped Breathing

The date was December 10, 2000. My condition had gone downhill rapidly, necessitating another admission to the hospital and another open lung biopsy. I was having difficulty breathing and my energy level was severely diminished. While x-rays and CT scans revealed obstructions in my lungs, an open lung biopsy was needed to determine if indeed it was still cancer (not infection, or scar tissue) that was causing the ever-increasing obstructions in my lungs. After the nurse wheeled me into the holding room (where patients waited until it was time to go into the operating room), we prayed for God's protection over me and wisdom and skill for the medical personnel, trusting in the Lord implicitly. A friend from church kept Daniel (who was 21 months old at the time) at their home while Linda waited with me in the holding room. While we waited, me lying on a gurney and Linda sitting next to me, I had no sense that this open lung biopsy would be any different from the first one. I felt completely at peace, completely relaxed.

We talked while we waited for the nurse to come get me. Linda and I chit-chatted about trivial things; we wondered how Daniel was doing at our friends' house, and Linda asked me what I wanted to do for my birthday (which was coming up in less than a week). God's peace was guarding our hearts and minds through Christ Jesus.

Back in May, the doctors performed an open lung biopsy to determine what was wrong with me (that procedure went smoothly, with no complications). Although at this time I was doing worse overall, and my breathing was more strained, I thought this operation would go just as smoothly as the first. An open lung biopsy is essentially surgery, but since the first biopsy went so well, I had no reason to think this one would be any different.

When it was time for me to go in to the OR, the nurse started my IV drip, and had me count backwards from 100. "100, 99, 98," …. I had barely counted to 98 when I began to drift off into lala land, fully expecting to wake up in the serenity of the recovery room after the surgery. What I experienced next was more like a scene from a horror movie.

The next thing I knew, I was wide awake, on the table, in the

He Stopped Breathing

middle of the operating room, with bright lights blinding me and machine alarms going off all around me. I was aware of all these things, yet I was writhing back and forth on the table in indescribable pain.

"Daniel! Daniel! Daniel!" The doctor kept calling my name. I could not hear him; I could not answer. I was screaming, crying, begging, pleading, "Make it stop! Just make it stop! Get me out of here!" Pain: excruciating pain: the most intense pain I have ever felt. Alarms were blaring, medical personnel were frantically scuttling around, and the doctor was standing over me trying to get me to answer (to make sure that I was stable and coherent). "What happened? Why am I lying awake on the operating table, writhing in pain? Why am I in such pain? What went wrong?"

Apparently, because of the severe congestion of my lungs (due to the advanced spread of the cancer) and the trauma to the body caused by the operation, I had stopped breathing on the table. The medical staff had to stop the anaesthetic, revive me and make sure I was stable before they could start the IV painkiller. Once I was stabilized, they started the IV painkillers, and I drifted off into a drug-induced haze. All of this probably lasted less than a minute, but to me it seemed like an eternity. The cancer tried to take me, but God said, "Not Yet!

Sometimes, when a person dies, their bowels and bladder empty out. Apparently, this happened to me on the table when I stopped breathing, and I had to be cleaned up after the procedure. Because of the complications with the biopsy, I had to stay in ICU for about a week. I was stable, but I had initially run a fever of 105, and had just stopped breathing in the middle of an operation, so I was kept in ICU until my condition was upgraded. ICU was not a pleasant experience. The unit I was in was essentially a large room, with four or five beds arranged in a circle, with no privacy (save for curtains hung from tracks in the ceiling that could be pulled around the bed). When you are in ICU, getting up and going to the bathroom is not an option. You do your business at the bed in a bed pan or jug. I have always been a little shy about peeing in front of people, so this was difficult for me. In fact, at the time, it was impossible; I was unable to go. Since holding it for too long could cause problems, a catheter would have to be used on me. I had never experienced a catheter before, so I asked the nurse if it would be painful. She said it was uncomfortable, but that it would not hurt. I made the mistake of believing her. Can you say painful!? Why do doctors and nurses lie about pain? Do they think that it will be easier on the patient if you are not expecting pain?

The results of the biopsy confirmed what the doctors suspected: the thing that was causing the obstruction in my lungs was still cancer, and it had spread. The treatment was not working. After spending several days in ICU, I was transferred to a standard room. So what now? Obviously, the chemotherapy was not working. I had gotten worse, not better…significantly worse. What would become of me? Would they try something different? More chemotherapy? Give up? Was the cancer going to win? Was this the end for me?

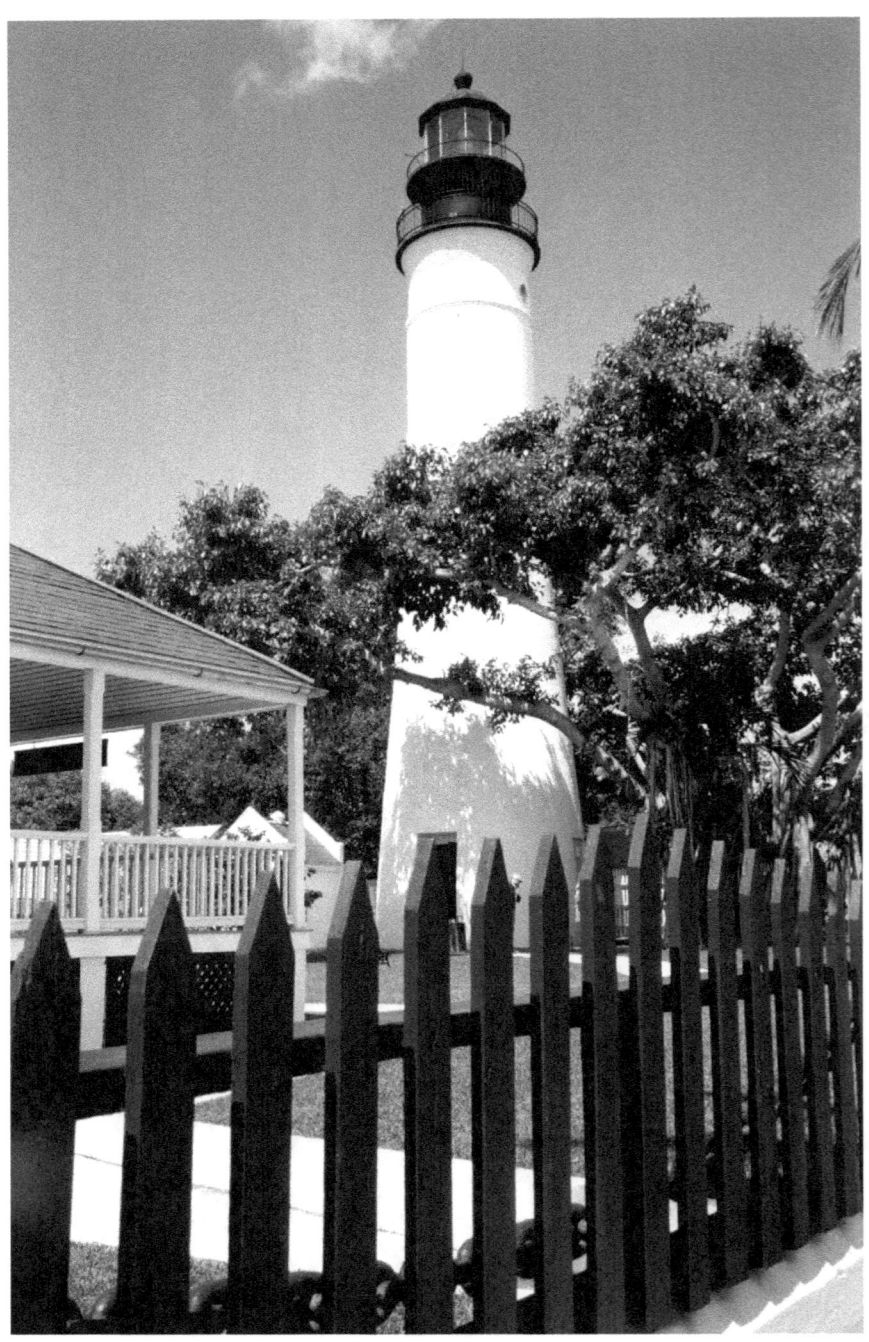

Chapter 2

The Salad Days

Who was Daniel Neff? Daniel was a warm, intelligent, good-looking young man who did not believe he was any of these things. He was a very good student in high school, and after graduation, he went on to college at Va Tech (Virginia Polytechnic Institute and State University) in Blacksburg, VA. At that time, he had no idea what he wanted to be, so he did not buckle down and study like he should have. He ended up dropping out during the first quarter of his second year at Tech. Some people are not ready for college right out of high school. In our society, we tend to have this mentality that everyone who has the grades and aptitude for college, should go straight to college from high school. This is a mistake. Anyone who does not have a clear vision of what they want to do when they finish high school, should get a job or join the military or serve in the Peace Corps. Something else to consider is the fact that after twelve consecutive years of schooling, some people need a break, before immersing themselves into four (or more) years of intense schooling. Okay, enough about that, I will save my dissertation on education for another book.

After spending about a year living with my parents and working the graveyard shift stocking groceries, I was well motivated to commit to a goal and work for it. If I had worked at a grocery store for a year or two right after high school, then went to college, I would have been motivated to focus on a goal and finish with a degree. I knew that I did not want to work in a grocery store for the rest of my life, but I did not have an academic path set out for college, so I decided to give air traffic control a try (following in my father's footsteps). I enlisted in the Air Force for the experience, with the intention of getting a job as an air traffic controller with the FAA in the civilian sector after completing my four-year commitment.

The Air Force was a great experience. I highly recommend the military to anyone. I developed a sense of honor and commitment that I lacked previously. I developed a lot of self-confidence, and the experience brought out many talents I did not know I had.

The Salad Days

I had many adventures during my time in the Air Force.

Basic Training was a great experience. It would be a stretch to say it was fun, but I would not trade it for anything in the world. Air Force Basic Training is conducted at Lackland Air Force Base in beautiful San Antonio, Texas, home of the Riverwalk. I did not get to see San Antonio, The Riverwalk, or any other local attractions, all I got to see was the confines of Lackland AFB: my barracks, our drill pad, and the mess hall. But I was not there for a vacation. I was there to be shaped into a young airman. The time-tested technique of tearing you down and building you back up really works. I was a shy, insecure young man when I enlisted in the Air Force, but by the time I finished Basic Training, I was confident and assertive. I became a squad leader and I began developing leadership qualities I did not know I possessed. The camaraderie in the military is another invaluable aspect of my experience; it is something I have not experienced anywhere else in life. Good old boys and tough guys from New York; Black, White, Hispanic and Asian; Christians, Jews, Muslims and non-believers: everyone worked together and got along. Racism and prejudice were not tolerated in the Air Force and the team concept was central. If one of the members of the squad failed, everyone failed. One of the objectives we had to pass (in order to complete Basic Training) was running a mile, in formation, within a given time limit. If one airman dropped out and failed to finish on time, everyone failed. One of the members of our squad struggled mightily to finish the run in the time allotted. John was not terribly out of shape or lazy, he was just not very athletic. We knew that if John could not complete the run, the whole squad would fail, so when it came time for our official run, a couple of us flanked him on the back line, locked arms with him, and "carried"

9

him through the run (we did not physically "carry" him, it was more a case of pulling him along.) As a squad, we pulled together and came up with a plan to get past this obstacle that stood in our way. It was the epitome of teamwork. That is something I will never forget.

Altus Air Force Base, my first assignment, was out in the middle of nowhere. (Southwest Oklahoma, near the Texas Panhandle.) Okay, Altus was not the end of the earth, but you could sure see it from there. Since Altus was 2 ½ hours from the nearest airport of any size (Will Rogers World Airport in Oklahoma City), I had to take a small commuter plane from Will Rogers Airport to the local county airport. As the puddle jumper (small 4-8 seat commuter plane) soared over the town of Altus en route to the municipal airport, bouncing in the clear air turbulence, I recalled the words of my instructor at Keesler Air Force Base, when he learned I was going to Altus, "you'll love Altus, there's a girl behind every tree." As I surveyed the landscape, looking for the girls behind the trees, I began to cry. Altus was flat, dry, and it seemed there were only half a dozen trees in the whole county; not exactly an encouraging start to my Air Force career. The population of Altus, without the military personnel, was less than 10,000. Hey, it was small, but it was backwards. I kid; Altus was a fun little town, and the people were great. Every Friday or Saturday night you could cruise from Walmart on one end of town, down to Sonic on the other end of town, then turn around and head back to Walmart. Then do it all over again, and again, and again. Ah, good times!

Southwest Oklahoma is very flat. You can see for miles and miles, and the sunsets are nothing short of spectacular, but being

The Salad Days

reared in Northern Kentucky I have always been partial to mountains. The flat lands of Southwest Oklahoma took some getting used to, but it was not completely hopeless: although Altus (and the surrounding county) was very flat, 15 miles to the north and about 50 miles to the east, there were a few small mountain ranges (technically, they are probably just hills, but mountain sounds cooler). The mountains (hills) to the north of Altus surround Lake Altus: a medium sized lake that provided a variety of recreational opportunities. Fishing, water skiing, hiking, camping and picnicking were enjoyed nearly all year round.

My buddies and I enjoyed hiking in the mountains (hills) around Lake Altus. Rattlesnakes are very common in Oklahoma, but especially in rocky, mountainous (hilly) terrain. The highest mountain (hill) near Lake Altus had some radio towers and a couple of buildings at its peak, and one day, a group of us decided we needed to make a trek to the peak. It seemed like a great adventure, to see what was at the top, what the view was like. It would be two to three hours up and a couple back down, we figured, easily doable in one day. The surface consisted of mostly large rocks (about the size, length and width, of a Volkswagen Bug) with small areas of dirt and grass in between at some points. I was leading the expedition up the hill; rambling along without a care in the world, not even thinking about wildlife, when all of a sudden, as I was about to step off a rock onto a dirt and grass spot, I was frozen by a very distinct sound, that of a rattle. Rattlesnakes, as the name implies, have a rattle at the end of their tail. When threatened, they will shake their tail, causing the characteristic rattle, in an attempt to ward off the predator. It worked. After gathering my composure, I informed my buddies that it might be best for us to cancel the expedition and head back down the mountain. None of my buddies shared this sentiment, since at that point, we were better than halfway to the top. Because of their desire to reach the peak (and the fact that they had not just had a close encounter of the rattling kind), my buddies decided that we were going to continue on our quest to the top of Rattlesnake Mountain (that's not the real name of the mountain (hill), but I don't remember the name and Rattlesnake Mountain sounds cool). In the course of his diatribe on the moral imperative of completing our quest, my friend Jim (who I remain close friends with even now), had made his way a little farther up the hill, bypassing the route I had taken, apparently operating on the assumption that the snake I almost stepped on was the *only* rattlesnake on Rattlesnake Mountain. Jim was chiding me on my lack of courage and resolve, making comments apparently meant to question my manhood, when he stopped in the middle of a sentence, uttering some choice words (I believe he said, "shucky-darn"). Jim was standing three feet away from one rattlesnake, and had just walked by another (almost stepping on it). Jim announced that after further consideration, he agreed with me that we should turn back. I guess I was not the only coward in the group. So we headed back to our cars; intrepid explorers we were not.

On another one of our hikes, on a different mountain (hill) in the Lake Altus region (Cave Mountain, again a made-up name), we discovered a small cave. There was an opening on either end, and a crevice at the top. We discovered the cave on a day hike, but we realized that it would be a cool place to hang out at night (there was no nightlife to speak of in Altus, aside from cruising up and down Main Street.) Frequently on our night off in the winter months, a group of us would go out to the lake, hike to the cave, and just hang out. One person would bring some beer, another would bring a boom box, and someone would bring a couple of Duraflame logs. We would build a fire using the Duraflame logs to stoke some Mesquite wood we found nearby, play some music, drink beer and enjoy the camaraderie. The air was crisp and clear, and the night sky, far away from any city lights, was amazing; the stars were too numerous to count.

As spring unfurls, melting away inhibitions, young men's hearts turn to thoughts of stripping down to their underwear and jumping into Lake Altus from a rock outcropping. Okay, that is not exactly how it unfolded. One day, one unseasonably warm day in late February, we were hanging out at the lake. The temperature was in the upper 60s, and after hiking for a while, we were kind of hot. So we figured that a leap into the lake would be refreshing. I never said we were rocket scientists; we were air traffic controllers. (I guess it is kind of scary to think that we were the ones responsible for making decisions to keep airplanes from flying into each other.) We found a rock that jutted out over the lake far enough to let down into deep water. Then we stripped down to our boxers, and proceeded, one by one, to jump off the rock into the lake. I need to pause here to explain a fact that some may not understand (my buddies and I definitely did not understand); water temperature takes a lot longer to warm up than air temperature. It takes weeks of warm weather (maybe months) for the temperature of the water in a large lake to warm up. So, while the air temperature might have been comparable to late May, the water was still February temperature. Cold. Very cold. Freezing cold. Imagine filling up a swimming pool with ice water, actual ice cubes and water, then jumping in. The water was so cold that as soon as I hit the water, I imagined myself popping up out of the water and scattering across the surface back to the shore like a cartoon character. Of course, despite seeing your buddy shrieking like a little girl as he swam back to the shore, leaving a wake like a boat behind him, we each had to go through with this leap of lunacy, lest we be labeled a sissy. Again, we were not rocket scientists.

Altus AFB had KC-135 refueling tanker aircraft (among other types). Being an air traffic controller, I got to ride along on a familiarization flight on one of the refueling missions. It would be a great opportunity to observe in-flight refueling operations. However, I was a little nervous about going on one of these flights. The runway at Altus was very long, nearly three miles long. (As a matter of fact, we were one the emergency landing sites for the Space Shuttle.) The KC-135 tankers, when filled with jet fuel for refueling, were extremely heavy and struggled to get airborne, even with the long runway. A few years later, larger, more powerful engines were retrofitted to the KC-135 to give them the power they needed, but before the upgrade it was always a little nerve racking watching one (from the control tower) on takeoff roll, hoping it would get airborne before running out of runway. Imagine being on one of those tankers as it rolls down the runway.

From my seat on the plane, I could see out the window, to the side of the field where the control tower was, as well as all the parking areas and hangers. I was very familiar with the layout of the airport, as I was a controller in the tower and learned all these things and surveyed the field (from the tower) every day. As we rumbled down the runway in that mobile gas station with wings, I took note of different landmarks as we passed them: midfield turnoff from the runway, (halfway down the runway); the control tower, (about two-thirds down the runway); C-141 parking area, (three-quarters down the field). Are we going to make it? I had watched literally hundreds of tankers roll down the runway (in my days working in the tower), lift off without incident, and then return later after their training mission was completed. I had no rational reason to be afraid, and yet, it was very disconcerting, knowing that the end of the runway was fast approaching and our wheels were still on the ground. I was not a religious man back then, but you can believe I was praying that day. Thankfully, before we reached the grass at the end of the runway, we lifted off and began, very slowly and methodically, climbing into the sunny Southwest Oklahoma sky. One of the reasons the base was located in Altus was the weather. Altus was a training base for several different types of planes, so good weather is essential for much of the operations. Altus averaged 307 (out of 365) days of VFR weather (weather conditions that allow a pilot to fly visually, without any instruments) each year.

As we climbed upward and settled into our cruising altitude, I began to relax and enjoy the scenery. We flew over the Texas panhandle, New Mexico, Colorado, Kansas, and back to Oklahoma. Watching the varied terrain go by was fascinating: mountains, farms, rivers, towns. The patchwork quilt of farmlands in Southeast Colorado and Kansas was especially striking.

A refueling tanker has a long boom that extends down from the tail of the plane. The plane that is to be refueled flies up directly behind and below the tanker and positions his aircraft to join up with the boom. The boom is controlled by an airman on the tanker, who lies on his belly in the tail section, operating the controls to line up the boom with the receptacle on the plane being refueled. The boom operator's station had an extra pallet next to him, allowing another person to observe the operation. Watching an aerial refueling operation from that vantage point was a treat and a privilege; something not everyone gets to see. I was close enough to literally see the color of the pilot's eyes.

Another exciting experience that I was privileged to have was to be working in the control tower during an air show in which the Thunderbirds performed. For anyone who does not know, the Thunderbirds are the Air Force fighter jet demonstration team (similar to the Navy's Blue Angels). The Thunderbirds fly F-16s and do many stunts, individually and in formation. During the air show, the Thunderbirds have their own controller who takes over and directs the team from the tower. We made sure the airspace was clear before the show, and then handed the tower over to them. But we did get to stay in the control tower and observe. Watching the Thunderbirds perform is always exciting, but being up in the control tower and getting to hear the communications that go on between the team and their controller was very exciting.

Air Traffic Control was a great job to have in the Air Force. I worked indoors in a climate-controlled environment: heat in the winter and air conditioning in the summer. I got to sit down most of the time, and I had one of the most exciting jobs in the Air Force (other than flying a plane). People talk about the stress of air traffic control, but I never felt any significant stress. I think the key is that you cannot dwell on the fact that a mistake could cause people to die (and millions of dollars in lost aircraft), while at the same time you have to remain cognizant of the fact that a bad decision could mean lost lives. It is not that I did not care that people could die if I made a mistake, I was just oblivious to it; I never thought about it. I took to air traffic control like a duck takes to flight. In technical training school at Keesler AFB, I was a natural, graduating a week early. At Altus, I checked out in minimum time, I was frequently relied on to handle the heaviest traffic periods, and I was the youngest, lowest ranking airman to check out in the Tower Coordinator position (a controller who would coordinate between the primary controllers in the tower and the radar approach control facility). I received many letters of appreciation and accommodation from pilots and wing commanders. When my enlistment was about up (about six months out), I applied to the FAA, and was offered a job. I then applied for an early out from the Air Force, received approval, and I was discharged on May 4th and started classes at the FAA academy in Oklahoma City on May 9th, 1989.

It seemed everything was going my way. My plan to train as an air traffic controller in the Air Force and then get a job with the FAA fell right into place. I had everything I wanted and needed, or so I thought.

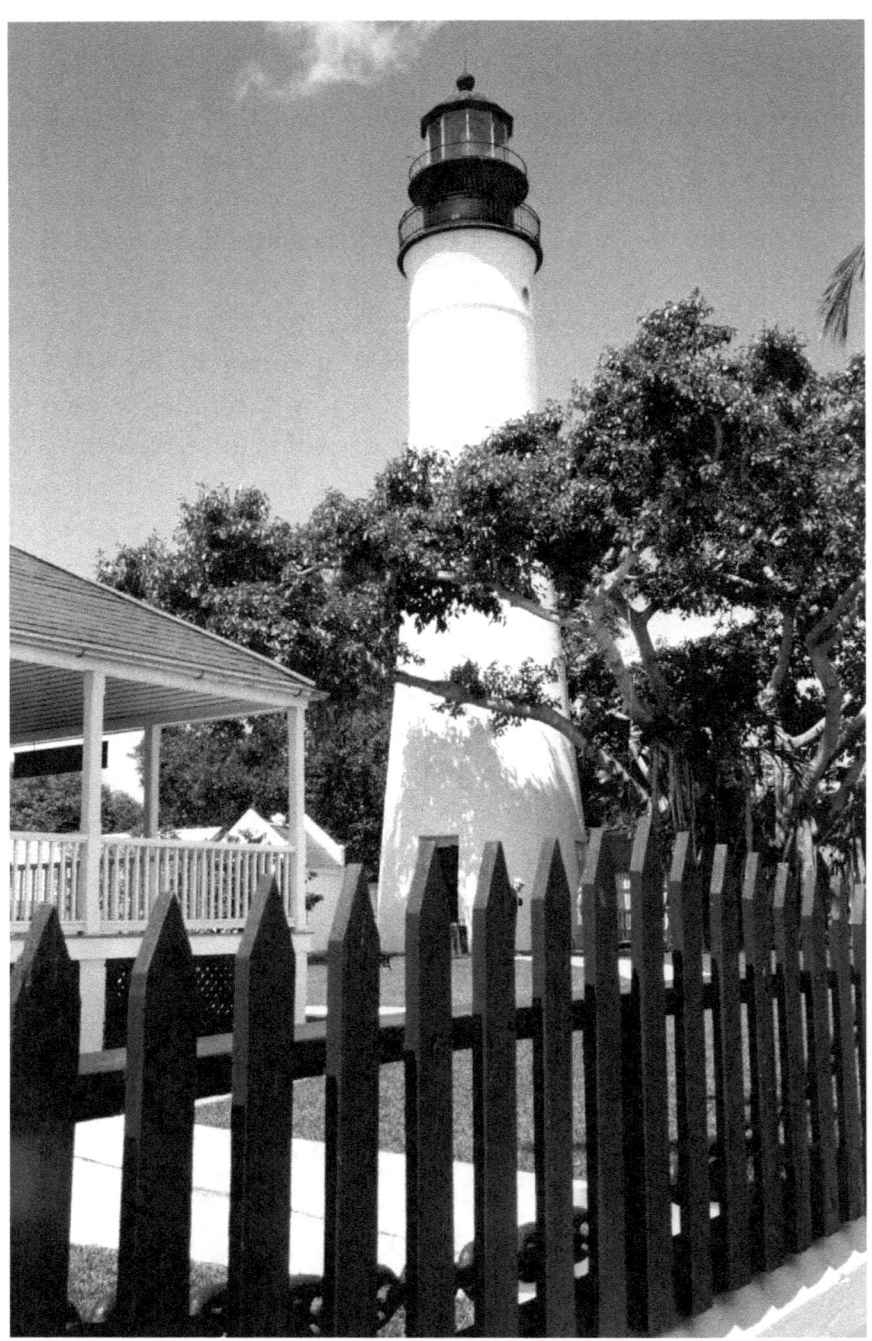

Chapter 3

Why Am I Here?

It was the summer of 1990, I was living in Colorado (a dream of mine for nearly 25 years), I had a very good job, and I was in good health. Still, something was missing. Despite having success in my life, I felt empty inside.

After spending four years in the Air Force as an air traffic controller, I got hired by the FAA, went through the FAA Academy in Oklahoma City and graduated near the top of my class (only outscored by an individual who had washed out of the

Academy previously and was on his second go-around). Upon graduation, I got my choice of going to Denver Center, Salt Lake Center or Seattle Center.

Ever since I visited Colorado as a twelve year old in the summer of 1976 (with my family), I was in love with the Rockies and wanted to live there more than any other place. I was awestruck by the beauty and majesty of the Rocky Mountains. I had been to the Smokies in the southeast, but the Rocky Mountains were a whole other world. Between the panoramic views, the soaring peaks, and the endless skies, I was smitten. Colorado was unlike any place I had ever been (and my family had traveled extensively when I was young). I had been to Toronto, Ontario, Niagara Falls, the Smoky Mountains, Myrtle Beach, Disney World, Key West, the NASA Space Center in Houston and many other destinations. My parents, Sally and Sonny Neff, were blessed, and they blessed us (my sisters, my brother, and me) with many great trips and memories.

My impression of Colorado did not leave me over the next 14 years. We moved from Oklahoma to New Jersey, then to Georgia briefly before my enlistment in the Air Force. I went to San Antonio, TX for basic training, to Biloxi, MS for technical training school, and then to my duty assignment in Altus, OK. I would listen to a certain song about the Rocky Mountains and dream of being in the Rockies. When I finished the FAA academy and had the opportunity to choose Denver Center, my longtime dream was finally coming true.

In the summer of 1989, I moved to Longmont, Colorado and started training at Denver Center. Longmont was nestled right up at the base of the foothills of the Rockies. I could jump in my car and be high up in the mountains in less than an hour, cruising down a twisty two-laner through a verdant mountain valley. I would take a picnic lunch with me and park at one of the scenic picnic areas. Nestled among the mighty pine trees, enjoying the mountain scenery and breathing in the clear mountain air, I was in paradise.

I have loved snow skiing since I first learned to ski in New Jersey as a 15 year old. Living in Colorado, I was able to go skiing every week on my day off. I had my choice of several top-notch ski resorts: Keystone, Breckenridge, Copper Mountain and Winter Park were all less than two hours from Longmont. I was in skier's heaven. In addition to recreational opportunities galore, the weather in Colorado was perfect for me. I do not do well in high humidity; Colorado is nearly devoid of humidity. The air is clear and the seasons mild. Colorado was a perfect place for me. I had nearly everything I could want or hope for, yet still I was empty inside.

I knew the one thing I did not have that I really wanted was a family. I was convinced that a wife and children would fulfill me, complete me. I had known since the first time I became interested in girls that I wanted to get married and have kids. The bachelor life never held any allure for me. Being alone, free to date every woman in town was not my idea of paradise. Perhaps if I looked like Brad Pitt or Patrick Swayze, I would have felt differently, but women were not exactly beating down my door. I wanted to settle down, have kids and have a house with a white picket fence: live the American dream. I was 26 years old at the time I moved to Colorado; I had no prospects for marriage, so I was getting very restless.

God Said Net Yet!

While living in Longmont, I met a really nice girl named Jennifer and we started dating. I was sure that I had found "the one". Jennifer was beautiful, smart, and we enjoyed each other's company. Well, to make a long story short, it did not work out. I was devastated. (While at the time I thought it was this one relationship with Jennifer that I needed, I would come to realize that I was looking for a mate to fill the void inside of me that no person can fill.) I quit my job, left Colorado, and moved back in with my parents in Georgia. My parents were thrilled! The one thing that was missing from their lives (living in a golfer's paradise, Peachtree City, GA, with no kids at home), was an out of work twenty-something-year-old son living in their spare bedroom, eating their food, and running up their electric bill.

I could not let go of my desperate need for a mate. I was still obsessed with the feeling that I had to have someone in my life to ease the pain of loneliness. Out of desperation, in an attempt to win back the love that I thought was the answer, I drove halfway (more actually) across the country to plead my case with Jennifer. Although I was very persistent, I did not stalk her, and I was respectful, and when she refused to see me unless I met with the campus chaplain at the same time, I knew she would never want the same thing I wanted. When she rejected me, I thought there was no point in going on. I had been in several relationships in the past that ended in disappointment, but this was the last straw. I felt like there was no point in trying anymore. I was sooo old (26), I could not wait any longer for someone to share my life with. I did not want to go on. While I never did actually attempt suicide, I did think about it; I even considered what method I might use. I actually thought that a wife was what I was missing and desperately needed. Soon it would be revealed to me what it was that I was missing, what it was I was looking for, what it was I really needed.

For years, through acquaintances and friends and coworkers, God had been gently revealing Himself to me, calling me to Him, to surrender my life to Him and serve Him. I resisted, I ran, I hid...but the Lord continued to pursue me. No matter how far or fast I ran, God patiently tracked me and continued to call me. I continued to reject Him. Something had to give, and it was not going to be God. One day, while driving down a road near Peachtree City, Georgia, I was listening to Charles Stanley, the famous Southern Baptist preacher, on the radio. He was talking about Jesus and His love for us, that He died on the cross to save us from our sins. I finally decided to give up the running. I was running away from God and towards things that can never truly fill that emptiness inside. As I was driving down the road that October day in 1990, I surrendered my will to His will. I dropped to my knees (figuratively, in my mind and heart, as I was still driving down the road), told God I was tired of running from Him, and that my life was His to do with as He pleased. I surrendered my heart and my life to Jesus, I have never been the same, and I have never regretted that life-changing decision. I found fulfillment for my emptiness; my hope comes from God.

The anxiousness, the fear, the emptiness that had haunted me for years melted away. I finally found that thing I had been looking for: peace in my soul, an eternal purpose that filled the void, which I had tried to fill in so many different ways. I have heard it described that we all have a God-shaped void inside of us, and nothing but a faith in Jesus can fill that void: no person or mate can fill it; no amount of money or power can fill it; none of

God Said Net Yet!

the pleasures of this world can fill the void inside of us.

John 3:16, 17

For God so loved the world that He gave His only begotten Son,

that whoever believes in Him should not perish but have everlasting life.

For God did not send His Son into the world to condemn the world,

but that the world through Him might be saved.

That is the Christian faith in a nutshell. From the moment I surrendered my life to Jesus, I knew I was supposed to be in some type of full-time ministry. I was certain I was not called to be a pastor or priest, and I did not feel called to be a foreign missionary. I always enjoyed working with youth, so the obvious initial thought was, "I should be a youth pastor". I volunteered with youth groups at the churches I was involved with, and later on I tried a couple of stints as a youth pastor. The first was a non-paid position in a start-up church. The second was a part time position in a church with 20-30 regular youth members. During this time, I spent a lot of time with youth, went with our youth group on a mission trip to Jamaica, coached softball, supervised lock-ins, and taught and mentored youth. There were some wonderful times: like the mission trip to Jamaica, and the ski trip to West Virginia (and making angels in the snow in our bathing suits just outside the swimming pool at the hotel), and there were heart wrenching times: like the funeral of Nathan, a teenager in the youth group who died in a car accident. While it was difficult, mourning his loss, it was a blessing to see how many kids Nathan influenced for Christ. There were many, many kids at the funeral, and at least one of them asked Jesus into His heart that day because of the impact Nathan had made on him.

While I enjoyed working with youth I always felt frustrated because I felt like I could not make a difference in their lives (since I only got to spend a couple of hours a week with them). This, of course, is not to say that youth pastors do not make a difference (they certainly do), it is just that my calling was not to be a youth pastor (if it was, I would have been content in that role).

During this period of my life, I lived with my parents for several years after leaving Colorado and my job with the FAA. It was a fruitful time in my life, but it was time to move on. My parents did not push me at all, they were very patient; however, I was concerned that they were growing weary of me living there. I was listening to a local call-in radio show, when a man called in saying that if his 26 year-old son Manny did not move out soon, he was going to have to kill him. I was 26, and my name is Daniel, or Danny. This was probably just coincidence, but it did give me pause. Living in my parents' house, with no bills, gave me a chance to get back on my feet. It also gave me an opportunity to spend quality time with my parents at a stage in life when most people are raising a family or living the single life. I had ample time (and latitude, thanks to the long-suffering benevolence of my parents) to take stock of my life, grow a little, and figure out where I was going next.

It just so divinely happened that some friends from church, Guy and Diane, lived on 20 acres in Roscoe, Georgia, in an old house they were restoring. On the property sat a doublewide trailer that was empty. Diane's mother had lived there until she died a few years prior. They wanted someone to live in the trailer and keep it up, in exchange for doing some chores around the property on the weekend. I jumped at the opportunity.

Roscoe (which happens to be the same name as my wife's grandfather) is a small community in the country just north of Newnan, Georgia. Newnan is a small city about an hour southwest of Atlanta, Georgia. Atlanta is a big city that is about....well, you probably know where Atlanta is. What is the old joke? When you die, on your way to heaven, you have to change planes in Atlanta. Guy and Diane's property was located on beautiful rolling hills in the Western Georgia countryside. There were two fenced off horse pastures of about five acres each, and a small, 2 acre pond that had been stocked with largemouth bass (but not fished very often, if at all. The bass were as big as my dog. Okay, maybe that is the fisherman in me exaggerating, but there were plenty of big bass in that pond; I know because I caught more than a few of them.) I would have free reign of this little piece of heaven.

I have always loved dogs, but had not had one since I was a teenager. I was not able to have a dog while I lived with my parents; they are not exactly dog people, and my dad was allergic. Therefore, one of the first things I wanted to do, after moving out to Roscoe, was get a dog. I had wanted a German Shepherd for a long time, so I was planning to get a German Shepherd. I had never bought a purebred dog before, so I was not aware of the cost; if I had known what the cost was, given my financial situation, I would not have planned on a German Shepherd. As it would turn out, my plans would be changed for me anyway. A couple of weeks before I moved in, a stray dog showed up on Guy and Diane's property. This was another divine occurrence. He was a beautiful young Golden Retriever, light in color and smart as a whip… He had a plain leather collar on, but no identification. It was clear that he had belonged to someone, but it was unclear whether he was lost or abandoned. Guy and Diane, being the good souls that they are, tied him up and started feeding him. They took care of him, put an ad in the local paper, and a notice with the local vet. No one claimed this beautiful dog, and Guy and Diane already had all the pets they could stand, so I got to keep him. A place of my own, lots of land to explore and fish to catch, and a wonderful companion to keep me company; I had not sought any of these things. Serendipity had visited my life, in the form of God's blessings.

Dusty, as I would name him, even though he was not a German Shepherd (the kind of dog I thought I wanted), was the best dog I have ever had. Linda always referred to Dusty as my "angel dog." Bobby Kelley, a friend of mine in Maine, used to tell me, "You'll never find another one like him". Dusty was a sweet dog. When Daniel was born, and we brought him home from the hospital, from the very beginning Dusty just knew how to behave around him. We held Daniel close to him, and Dusty would smell him and gently kiss him. Dusty always knew to be gentle around Daniel, and as Daniel grew and began to crawl and later walk, we never had to worry about Dusty stepping on Daniel or knocking him down; he was as careful as a loving parent. When Daniel was three, Dusty would lay in the grass in the back yard, chewing on a stick, and Daniel would lay on Dusty's back, chewing on a stick too. This of course thrilled his mommy!

When I worked weekends at a boys ranch in Georgia, I would

take Dusty with me. One day, somehow Dusty ended up loose in the yard with a young, three legged deer. This deer was one of the animals in the wildlife rescue program at the ranch (it had been hit by a car and lost a leg, and was nursed back to health as part of the program). Dusty took off after the deer and my heart jumped; I thought for sure that deer was a goner. However, Dusty, in his amazing way, knew not to hurt the deer. Dusty would chase the deer until he caught up to it, then lie down and wag his tail. Then, when the deer got a little further away from him, Dusty would give chase again. When he caught back up to the deer, again Dusty would lay down behind him, and never laid a paw on him or tried to bite him. I believe Dusty was trying to boost the deer's confidence that he was still a great running deer.

One day, when we were working at a group home in Maine, in a girls cottage, Dusty performed an amazing act of sensitivity and compassion unlike anything I have ever seen. One of the girls (I will call her Cindy) was sitting at the table, sobbing as she recalled a very painful memory. Dusty walked up to her, put his head in her lap, and looked up at her, as if to say, "I'm here for you." (This was not something that Dusty did very often, if ever.) He was truly an angel dog, and as Bob said, "I will never find another one like him."

In addition to the cottage program we were in (which was set up to be like a normal home), there was another program (staff-enhanced) on campus that had around-the-clock awake staff for kids with more intense issues. Part of their daily routine included a walk around the part of the campus we lived on. The rules about pets were pretty lax, so we were able to let Dusty outside, off the leash, to roam freely. He would routinely join the staff-enhanced group on their daily walks. All of the kids and the staff in this program knew Dusty and kind of felt that he was their dog.

Being in Maine, the winters were long with lots of snow that would cover the ground for months. It was like living in the middle of a Norman Rockwell painting. Although I had been a snow skier for many years, I had never taken the opportunity to learn how to cross country ski. I finally took up the skinny skis in Maine, with a 2400 acre campus (much of it wooded) right out my back door to explore. Dusty loved to accompany me in treks through the woods. I loved his company, but most times I ended up having to take him back to house after a little while. Dusty would follow so closely behind me that he would repeatedly step on the back of my skis and slow me down. In addition, the snow would start to freeze and clump up between his claws, causing him to stop and pull at the clumps with his teeth. In spite of what you may see in some kids' movies, Golden Retrievers would not make good sled dogs.

Dusty passed away in November of 2008, at the ripe old age of 14 (98 in dog years). The date was November 5, 2008, a Wednesday. If the date sounds familiar, that is because it is an historic date in American history. On Tuesday, November 4, 2008, for the first time in the history of the nation, America elected an African-American, Barack Obama, as its president. Either Dusty thought, "I am an old dog, I have lived to see the election of the first African-American president; I can die now"…or he thought, "I do not like the liberal direction this country is taking, I have lived a good long life; it is time to give up the ghost." I will let you decide. Dusty had developed a seeping wound, was on antibiotics for the injury, and he was very lethargic. He was lying on the floor in the living room, looking very tired, and breathing heavily. I went into the other room to work on the computer for a while. When I came out, I knew as soon as I saw Dusty that he was gone. He was lying on his side, with his mouth wide open and his tongue hanging out, stiff as a board. I wept. Given Dusty's age, and his reaction to the medication, we knew that these might be his last days, but nothing prepares you, emotionally, for the passing of a beloved pet. They become a member of the family, and you become emotionally attached to them.

I went upstairs and told Linda and Daniel that Dusty was gone. It was hard to get the words out. Daniel was nine years old at the time. He had known Dusty all his life, from the day he came home from the hospital. Daniel is an only child, and in some respects Dusty was like a brother to him, so it was very hard on Daniel. Some people think you should shield children from the death of a pet, but we do not agree with that philosophy. Actually, mourning a lost pet is a great way for children to learn and practice a skill they will use throughout their lives. The three of us went downstairs and spent a few minutes with Dusty, told him that we loved him and that we would miss him. We each took turns. Watching Daniel kiss Dusty good-bye and tell him that he loved him was tough but encouraging. It was hard because it was obvious that his little heart was breaking. At the same time, I knew that Daniel was going through the grieving process and learning a valuable lesson about life and death. For the next month or so, in the evening as he wound down and got ready for bed, Daniel would cry over Dusty. It was a hard time for him, but grieving is not supposed to be easy. Dusty lived a long, happy life, and we miss him. We will never find another one like him. Since we were living on a property that did not belong to us, we decided to have Dusty cremated rather than burying him in the yard. So I wrapped up Dusty's stiff, lifeless body in a blanket, carried him to the car, laid him on the back seat, and drove him to the vet. The vet took care of the arrangements and notified us when the ashes were ready.

Young Dusty loved life there in Roscoe, GA in 1996; there was plenty of land and woods for him to explore and many deer to chase. Dusty would go off into the woods, exploring and chasing deer, and come back an hour later, looking like he was going to drop from exhaustion. One day, I was standing by a fence down by the fishing pond, and I saw, in a flash, a deer go tearing past me. A couple of seconds later there went Dusty, close on his trail. As far as I know, he never caught that deer, but it was not for lack of effort. There was a large patch of ground on the property, maybe a half an acre or so, that was covered in weeds about five feet tall; Dusty turned it into a playground. He would run into the middle of the weeds, and every 10 seconds or so, he would leap up into the air, putting his head above the tops of the weeds, in an attempt to figure out where he was. He would run a little more, and then pop up again. It brought joy to my heart to see him so happy.

While living in Roscoe, I worked in the construction field, building houses. I worked for Mr. Thompson, who owned a small construction company. There were five of us on the crew, me and four real characters: Travis, James, Steven "slobber-dog" and Hoss (not his real name, I do not remember it, but if you ever saw the TV show "Bonanza", you know what this guy was like). Travis loved to make fun of the way I talked, I guess because I talked normal English and they all spoke redneck. When they agreed with something you said, they would say "show-nuff" (a derivative of "sure enough"). I would try and try to say "show-nuff" but it would always come out as "sure enough". "Danno," Travis would say, "you crack me up.... *Sure enough* (mocking me with his emphasis on non-redneck speak)". I guess Travis was a fan of Hawaii 5-0, because he called me Danno *all* the time, and I must have heard the phrase "Book-em Danno" about a thousand times. I was happy to provide them with so much entertainment. I learned a lot about construction, but even more about people. There was never a dull moment.

On one particularly rainy, muddy day we loaded up the truck and went to town to eat lunch. We walked in the front door, over to the table the host led us to, and sat down. It felt good to be in doors, out of the chilly rain. Building houses gives you one heck of an appetite; this day was no exception. As we were sitting there, looking over our menus, I noticed one of the waiters looking at me and scowling. I had no idea why he was upset with me, until one of my coworkers directed my attention to the muddy trail leading from the front door to my chair. I realized that my boots were full of mud and I had neglected to clean them off. I felt bad about making such a mess, but I was really hungry so I did not give it another thought. We ordered lunch, wolfed it down and then headed back to work. Later that night, at home, I woke up in the middle of the night, violently ill. I will spare you the gory details, but suffice to say I thought I was I going to die. I do not know if it was coincidence, or if the cooks decided to pay me back for messing up their floor, but needless to say (I will say it anyway) I never ate at that restaurant again.

Although working as a carpenter was not exactly my life's

Why Am I Here?

dream, it was something to do, and it paid the bills. I was enjoying life in Roscoe, not really searching for anything, when God serendipitously interrupted my life again. One evening, while at dinner with our singles group from church, my life would change (in more ways than one). One of the members of our group, April, worked at a ranch in Warm Springs, Georgia (about an hour south of Roscoe) that provided a home for troubled teenagers. Some of the youth had been removed from their home by the state, while others just had nowhere to go. April informed me that this ranch was interviewing for a weekend, relief houseparent position. April knew that I loved working with kids. This position was for a single individual who would work with others on the weekend to provide time off for the full-time staff. I was very intrigued by this opportunity. I called the next day and they asked me to come down for an interview.

Warm Springs, GA is (at least in 1996 it was) a quaint southern town reminiscent of yesteryear. The shopping district is composed of hundred year-old brick buildings with wood columns and fabric awnings. The ladies speak with a slow, southern drawl and call you honey. Outdoor courtyard shops with gazebos and ivy-covered trellises invite guests to browse for gifts in the sweet, balmy southern air, while indoor shopping abounds for inclement weather and those who prefer air conditioning. Warm Springs is also home to FDR's Little White House and Warm Springs Institute for Rehabilitation.

Driving up to the ranch in Warm Springs evokes feelings of days gone by, when time moved more slowly and life was simpler. A large, rustic wooden sign hanging over the entrance to the ranch greets visitors as they drive up Bar Rest Ranch Road. Acres and acres of open pastures back up to wooded hills: Pine Mountain and Franklin D Roosevelt State Park to be specific. Dozens of horses roam the pastures which flank both sides of the long gravel drive leading up to the main buildings. I expected to be greeted by Grandpa Walton in overalls. It was an idyllic setting for a home for teenagers. In addition to the home for troubled teens, the ranch was home to a therapeutic horseback riding program and a wildlife rescue program. People with a wide range of disabilities, from spinal injuries to Down's Syndrome could benefit from the unique program; a program that allowed individuals to work muscles that they normally couldn't. The wildlife rescue program took in injured animals: from birds to deer, then nursed them back to health, and released them back into the wild, if possible. These were terrific programs in and of themselves, but they were especially beneficial because it gave the boys something to do and the boys were able to learn valuable new skills and derive a sense of purpose. Some of the boys shoveled out horse stalls, while others brushed the horses or prepared them for riding. Still others got to learn how to nurse injured animals back to health.

The lovely lady who interviewed me at the ranch for the houseparent position is now my wife. Little did I know she was interviewing me as a potential husband at the same time she was interviewing for the houseparent position (well, according to Linda she was not interviewing me as a potential husband. As she tells it, she had become frustrated with the whole dating game, and had come to the place in her life where she wanted to have a resume and be able to interview the next man she dated beforehand. Now she had my resume in hand, and knew just about everything about me). While she says she was only interviewing me for the houseparent position, I thought a couple of the questions were curious. I did not understand the relevance of whether I enjoyed long walks on the beach and antiquing. I did not see what those activities had to do with working with troubled teenagers, but I answered as best I could. I say all this in jest. Of course, she was not interviewing me as a potential husband, but it is funny that it worked out that way. Anyway, more on that story later.

I passed the interview (in both respects), was then interviewed by the director (who just so happened to be a retired air traffic controller), and was offered the job (the houseparent job that is, I had to work a little harder for the other job). During the first weekend working with the kids, I knew, I knew that this was my calling. I finally knew what I wanted to be when I grew up, now I just had to grow up (I was 32 at the time). My wife will tell you it has been a long process (which is not yet complete). The job was, for the most part, spending time with the kids, mentoring them, teaching the life skills they had missed due to their situation. We went fishing, camping, swimming. We played sports, watched movies, and cooked meals together.

One of the boys (I will call him Billy) made quite an impression on Linda and me. He was a good kid, with a good heart, and you could tell he really just wanted a family of his own. Once we started dating seriously, Linda and I talked of adopting Billy once we got married. We never did adopt Billy, but it probably would not have been a good idea for newlyweds, and once we had been married for a few years, he was 17 or 18, almost an adult. Over the years, we served as surrogate parents for dozens of kids. Some you have an impact on, others you do not. While you tell yourself you cannot reach them all, that was never a consolation to me, and I felt like I failed each kid that I was not able to help. Working with youth in a group home setting was a very different kind of life. It was great fun and very rewarding. Challenging yes, but also very rewarding. These kids are not bad kids, they just need to know someone cares, and they need a positive role model to show them the way.

Initially I continued to work my construction job while working at the ranch on the weekends. I would work all week on my construction job in the Newnan area, and then on Friday evening I would drive down to Warm Springs. After spending the weekend working with the boys, I would leave early Monday morning to meet my work crew with Thompson Construction Company, and start the cycle all over again.

From the moment we met, Linda and I were both strongly attracted to one another. However, because of our desire to observe professional decorum, neither one of us let our feelings show. After a few weeks working there, we finally had an opportunity to spend some time together. The ranch had tickets for the boys to attend an Atlanta Braves baseball game on a Wednesday night. The game was during the middle of the week, when I did not work. The rest of the staff from the ranch was away at a conference. Linda was filling in, supervising the boys. Linda and I would be the chaperones for the trip to the Braves' game, so we arranged to meet at an exit off the interstate near where I lived.

Why Am I Here?

(From Linda's point of view, in her voice)

I was very nervous about contacting Dan to go along as a chaperone, not wanting to seem forward. I called him and we made the arrangements about where to meet. Dan drove the van from the rendezvous point, and I sat on the bench seat (behind the driver and passenger seats) with some of the boys, my feet propped up on the snack cooler. As we made our way through South Atlanta on I-85, Dan turned and looked over his right shoulder to make a lane change. It hit me like hand bells ringing...my dream from that past February. {I dreamt that I was in a van full of teens, with my feet propped up on the cooler. "Greg Brady" was driving the van and turned back to look at me! We were to be married.} There I was, my heart stopped, trying to catch my breath, living out my dream, as Dan looked back at me and smiled! Dan favored Greg Brady at that time, curly hair and all with one dark eyebrow that stretched across his forehead. As he smiled and checked for traffic, I knew; this was the man I was to marry!

A couple of nights later, when Dan was at the ranch (filling in for the houseparents that were still away at the conference), after the boys went to bed, we had a chance to sit and talk. We finally had a chance to talk openly about how we were feeling about each other and share our dreams and goals. When I first asked him if we could talk, Dan thought I was evaluating his work and that he might be fired. Ha ha! Men! Within a week, Dan told me that he knew I was the one for him. I shared 'the dream' I had dreamt with him and how it had been fulfilled. I did not know how God could work it out though. We started dating and knew early on that we wanted to be serious. Very soon though, life would dictate that we would have to make a decision about how serious we were. I was preparing to move back home to Andalusia, AL the next month (May 1996) to help my father care for my mother (who was going through some difficult health issues). Dan said, "God will provide a way if this is really His plan for us."

Jeremiah 29:11 became our verse: we claimed it through our engagement, and on our wedding day, and through each chapter of our marital adventures. It would prove to be especially comforting when Dan was sick with cancer.

Jeremiah 29:11

For I know the thoughts that I think toward you, says the Lord, thoughts of peace and not of evil, to give you a future and a hope.

Why Am I Here?

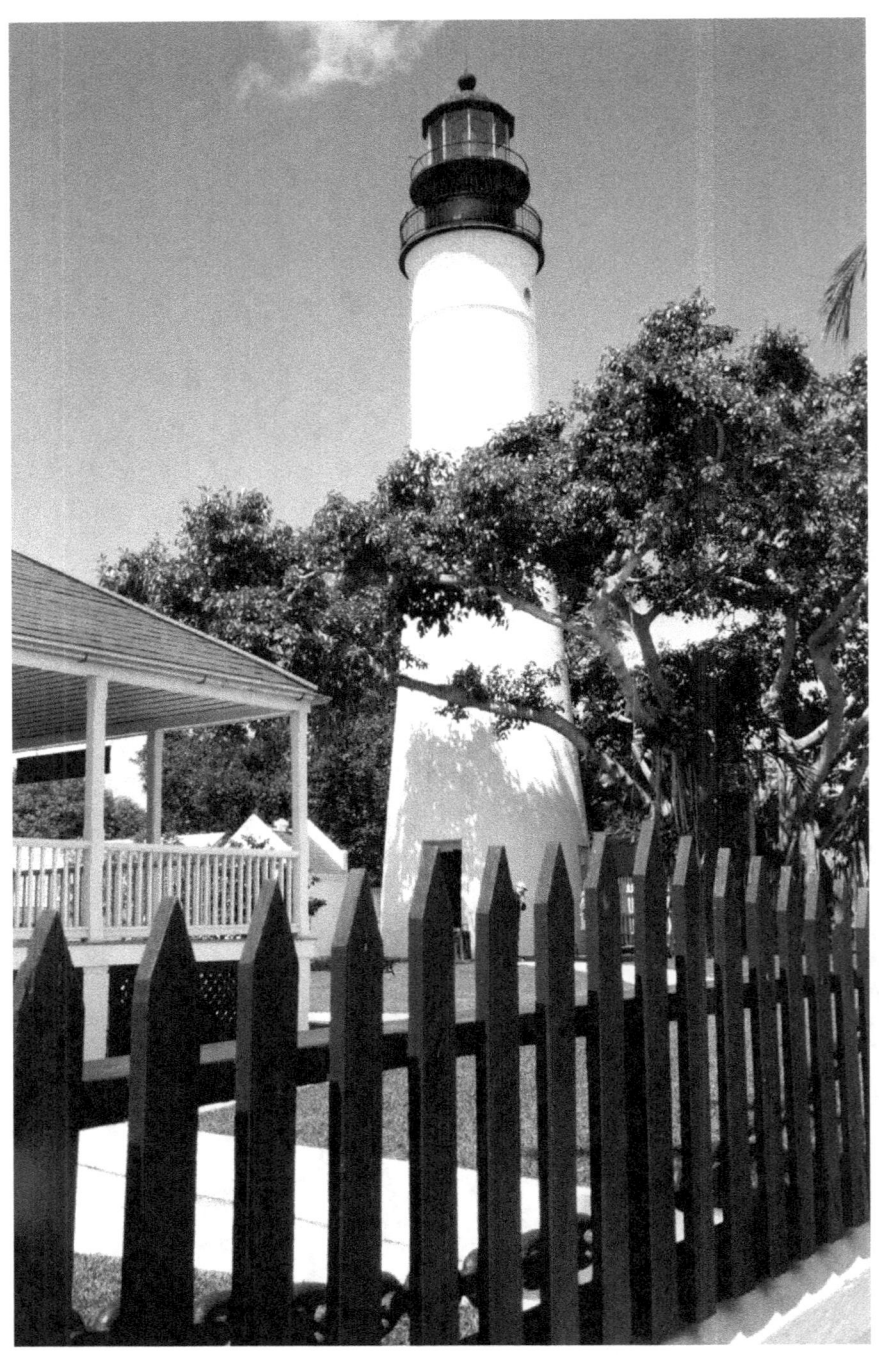

Chapter 4

Married With Child

In the beginning, our (Linda and I) desire to be together was tested acutely. Not only did we live an hour away from each other, but back home in Andalusia Linda's mother (Betty) was going through a very difficult ordeal. Betty had quadruple bypass heart surgery, and then a Staph infection set in that took months to be eradicated and took her right leg below the knee. Every weekend, Linda traveled home to Andalusia to be with her mother, and I worked at the ranch. During the week, while Linda was working in Warm Springs, I lived and worked an hour away. It is amazing that we were able to see each other at all, but love will find a way. About a month after we started dating, Linda decided she was going to leave her job at the ranch and move back to her hometown (Andalusia, Alabama...Roll Tide!) to help take care of her mother. Andalusia is about three and a half hours from Roscoe, GA, where I was living at the time. This presented a problem, since this move would require Linda to leave Warm Springs and therefore I would not see her unless I traveled to Andalusia. They, whoever "they" are, always say that long distance relationships do not work, so I was faced with a decision (because, of course "they" are never wrong).

I considered my full-time job and my living situation at the time to be transitory; I had no desire for either of these to be long-term situations in my life. While I enjoyed the work I was doing, and I loved living in the country in Roscoe, I knew that life held more for me than building houses and living all alone. Leaving Roscoe would be very difficult, but I would rather be anywhere with the woman I love than alone in a country paradise.

I knew Linda was the one, so I decided to move to Andalusia, rent a house, get a job and live there until we got married. Linda lived with her parents. We are old-fashioned, and we believe in waiting until marriage, so we did. I was able to continue commuting to the ranch to work on the weekends. It was a long drive, but I enjoyed working with the boys more than any job I ever had (even air traffic control). It was about a 3 ½ hour drive from Andalusia to the ranch, but the shift was from 10 PM Friday night to 8 AM Monday morning, so I only had to make the drive twice a week). After a few months, the long commute did get to be too much, and I had to stop, however I still knew that working with youth in a residential setting was my calling, and that one day in the future I would return to this work.

We lived in that small southern town as long as I could stand it, almost a whole week. I am not saying Andalusia is small, but a big night on the town is going to WalMart and then to Sonic for a milk shake (they now have a Super WalMart, WooHoo!). If it was a really special night, we would take in a movie at the vintage movie theater. The only movie theater in town, right in the middle of downtown, was a two-screen theater in an old brick building with a large neon marquee on the side of the building. It was the kind of theater you see in a movie about the 1940s or 50s. Andalusia is a really nice little town and the people are terrific. I should know I married one of them. Good, old-fashioned Americans who would do anything for you, real salt of the earth type people. Andalusia is actually a lot like a modern day Mayberry. If you do not know what Mayberry refers to, shame on you! Watch an episode of "The Andy Griffith Show." The town of Andalusia just did not suit me personally. The nearest town of any size (with a mall or Home Depot, was at least 45 minutes away). We lived there for a year and a half (which was longer than I could stand), then moved to Jacksonville, Florida.

Linda and I both loved working with kids, and while we were in Andalusia, we got involved in a program (that originated in Birmingham, Alabama) that targets troubled teens and their families. The program seeks to intervene in the lives of troubled youth when they just start to get into trouble, before they get deeply involved in criminal behavior, drugs, gangs, etc. Working with this population was at the same time frustrating and rewarding. At the end of the evening for the first few weeks of this nine week program (which consisted of a once-a-week meeting), we were on the verge of tears, feeling hopeless, feeling that our efforts were futile. As the weeks went by though, it was amazing to see God work in the lives of these families. We taught on subjects like trust and family relationships and substance abuse. We participated in fun exercises to illustrate the subject, and then broke off into small groups to discuss what we learned. There is nothing that compares to seeing broken lives transformed before your eyes and knowing that you played a small part in making it happen.

The real frustration of working with troubled youth is that in order to have support, both financial and even societal support, you have to have a complex, academically tested behavioral program in place. Take it from someone who has spent years in this field, the *only* thing that produces a real, lasting change in a troubled young person is the power of God and of prayer. A structured program of some sort is helpful to deal with negative behaviors, but the absence of the spiritual component (more specifically the absence of that spiritual component being God and being the absolute central component of the program) guarantees that most of the youth will fail. Linda and I worked in a program that had a symbol of the program's core mission belief. At the center was a boy, with the many aspects of life that are important, surrounding the boy. Among these was religion. While this symbol is a good starting point, I would say that the best formula would have God at the center, and portray that the youth's relationship to God would determine their success in every aspect of life. If the youth's relationship with God is broken, he will struggle in all areas of life. Of course, having one's relationship with God right does not automatically guarantee success in all areas of life, that requires diligence and dedication (whatsoever you put your hand to, do it with all your might), but it (one's relationship with God) is a good starting point.

At the time we were in Andalusia, there was an effort to start this same intervention program in Jacksonville, Florida as well, and we moved to Jacksonville with the intention of helping to get the program up and running. Rick, a very good friend of mine from my Air Force days lived in Jacksonville, and I had visited him many times. Therefore, I was already familiar with the city. Rick and his wife allowed us to stay with them until we found a place to live. Rick and Lori have two beautiful daughters who are grown now, but they were very young at the time. It was a blessing to live with them for a little while. I am six foot two, not a giant by any measure, but I guess I seem like one to a young girl whose father is shorter than average. (I am trying to be nice here. No, Rick is not a hobbit, but he is short. However, what Rick lacks in height, he more than makes up for in heart. Wow, what a cliché!) Anyway, one day Rick's daughter Katy (8 years old at the time) was playing over at a friend's house. A knock came at the front door, and I went to the door an opened it to see who was there. There stood Katy and her little friend, and Katy exclaimed to her friend, "See, isn't he huge!" You would think I was Andre the Giant. There must be something about my build that makes me look much taller than I am, because I remember my friend Russ used to joke that I was "freakishly" tall.

While the (at-risk teen) program fizzled in Jacksonville due to lack of support, we enjoyed our time there. Jacksonville is a great place to live. Jacksonville is the largest city, in terms of area, in the

U.S. The St. Johns River flows right through the middle of downtown Jacksonville. Jacksonville Landing, located on the river, has many restaurants and shops and an outdoor performance stage that hosts a variety of acts and events. You are never more than about 45 minutes from the beach. Jacksonville has an NFL football team, the Jaguars. There are several large, modern shopping malls, and many recreational options.

Two and a half years into our marriage (in 1999), while in Jacksonville, we had our son Daniel. Seeing the birth of my son was one of the most amazing, joyful experiences of my life; I highly recommend it to everyone. While your wife is pregnant, you know there is another life growing inside her, but to see that baby come out and then boom, there is another life in the world! Wow! I got to cut the umbilical cord, which was very difficult to cut even with sharp surgical scissors. If you have ever tried to cut anything with those safety scissors they use in kindergarten, you know what I mean. I think umbilical cords are used for the safety line (tether) which astronauts use when they go outside the space shuttle for repairs...seriously. Witnessing the miracle of birth is something everyone should do if they have the chance.

I got to change Daniel's first diaper in the hospital. It was one of those comical moments you normally see in the movies. I left Daniel lying on the bed and walked a few feet away to get a clean diaper (relax, at that age they cannot move or roll, so there was no danger of him rolling off the bed. Linda was sitting in a chair across the room). I was not looking directly at Daniel, but I heard a strange sound. About the time I realized it was some sort of liquid splashing on the floor, I looked over to see a stream of pee arcing up from Daniel, going about two feet in the air, and landing on the floor next to the bed. And Daniel was just a grinnin'. Ah, memories!

Between cultivating our marriage and having a child, not to mention the pesky task of working and paying bills, the mission of helping hurting teens in a residential setting got put on the back burner for a few years. We went to work, made some friends, got involved in our church, played at the beach, and explored Florida.

During the time we lived in Florida, we were blessed with the opportunity to travel and see many different cities and points of interest. From Panama City to Sarasota to Key West and Miami. In addition, there was Pensacola and Orlando and St. Augustine and Tallahassee. We visited Silver Springs in Ocala, Disney World and Sea World in Orlando, the Southernmost Point of the US and the Hemingway House and Mallory Square in Key West. Florida truly is a vacation paradise. No, the Florida Department of Tourism did NOT pay me to write this section.

St. Augustine, just south of Jacksonville is a marvelous town to visit, and was just a short drive from Jacksonville. I highly recommend it to anyone. St. Augustine is the oldest city and the oldest port in the continental United States. There are historic forts, bridges, lighthouses, lots of shopping, great dining, and beaches. St. Augustine is less than two hours by car from Jacksonville, Orlando and Daytona.

When our son Daniel was just three months old, he got to visit Disney World and Sea World. My family (parents, siblings and their children) got together for a Florida vacation. We took in Disney World, Dinner with Mickey and watching fireworks from the roof of the Contemporary Hotel. On another day, we went to

God Said Not Yet!

Sea World. During the show at the lakeside amphitheater, Daniel, at 3 months old, was featured on the Jumbotron during one of the shows.

One year we took a trip down the west coast of Florida from Tampa to Sarasota to Alligator Alley to Key West. We stopped in Sarasota to see the Cincinnati Reds in spring training (I have followed the Reds since I can remember, early '70s and this was the first time I got to attend Spring Training). We drove across Alligator Alley to Miami, and then down to Key West. We stayed in a campground in Sugarloaf Key, saw many sites, ate some great seafood, and met a family from Mentor, Ohio, who would become good friends.

Our life in Florida was very good; however, I was very dissatisfied in my work. I had a handyman business, and all my customers loved my work; but I was very frustrated. From a very young age, I was interested in architecture. I enjoyed drawing plans for buildings and airports and houses. Conceptualizing and drawing new creations always fascinated me. There were several times in my life when I had opportunity or desire to pursue this vocation, but never followed through. While in college at Virginia Tech in 1982-1983, I had a roommate who was in the architecture program. I got to visit the classrooms and studios. I hung out at his fraternity (primarily architects) and had the opportunity to get to know many young, aspiring architects. My interest was renewed, but I lacked confidence. I thought that architecture was too lofty a pursuit for me. I thought architecture was for really talented people, not me. I did not think I had what it took to be an architect, so I let it go. To this day, that is a regret of mine. I know (now) that I had the talent and passion to be a good architect. I know architecture is something I would have excelled at and a life I would have enjoyed. (Although I know now that God had other plans for me, the anguish of that broken dream still plagues me from time to time.)

In 1999 (at the age of 35), I decided it was time for me to pursue this dream. I was going to go for it, put all the doubts aside and pursue a career as an architect. I grew up in the greater Cincinnati, Ohio area, and always had a desire to return to that part of the country. When I found out the University of Cincinnati had an architecture program, I decided to apply for admission. I filled out the required paperwork, and we took a trip to visit the university. The thought of going back to Cincinnati and studying architecture in the Queen City was very exciting, as was the prospect of moving to a climate that actually had seasons. Some people like the endless summer of Florida; I am not one of those people. Florida has 11 months of heat, followed by a one month cold snap, then back to 11 months of hot, humid misery. I honestly do not know how anyone survived in places like Florida before air conditioning was invented. Cincinnati is located in part of the country that has four, distinct, beautiful seasons. It is a unique area in that the winters can seem as cold as Alaska, while summers are comparable to Death Valley. Autumn is my favorite season in Cincinnati. The temperatures could not be more pleasing. Most days are about 70 degrees, with little humidity, a light breeze, and ample sunshine. (That is how I remember it anyway.) And the colors: yellows, brilliant golds, vibrant shades of red and purple. The only place I have seen more beautiful fall colors is New Hampshire.

I was accepted to the University of Cincinnati and planned to

God Said Not Yet!

start my studies in the fall of 2000. It was the spring of 2000 and everything was set in motion for me to start school at UC and finally pursue this lifelong dream of becoming an architect.

My world was about to be turned upside down.

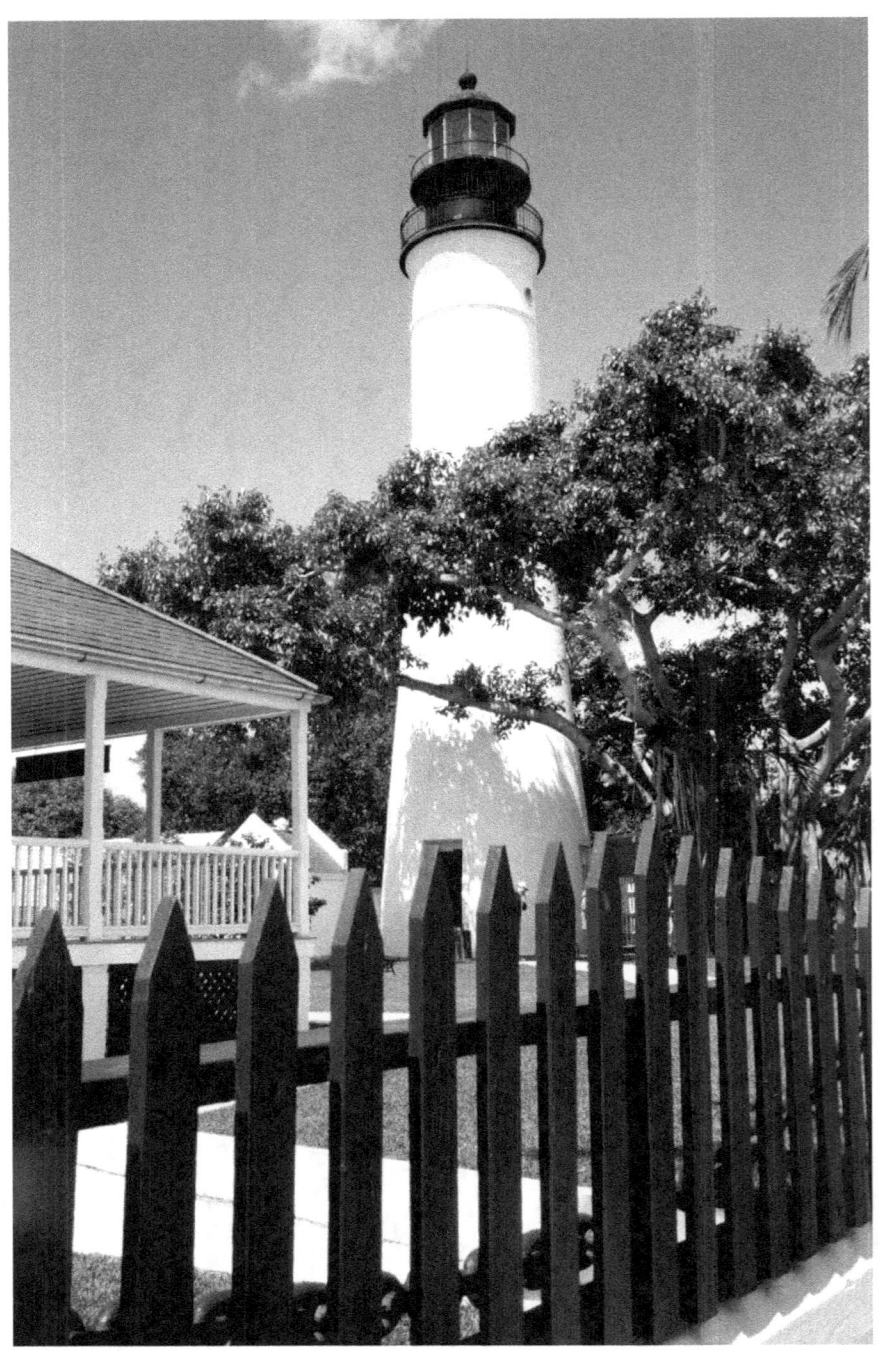

Chapter 5

Cancer, the Most Feared Word in the English Language

I always thought I was a healthy person. I kept myself in good shape. I was not a triathlete, but I kept active, playing softball into my 30s. I maintained a reasonably healthy diet. I usually ate whole grains, like whole wheat bread, fruits and vegetables, and never consumed more than 5 pounds of chocolate per day. I discovered that my diet was not all that healthy, but like many Americans I was misinformed and thought, believed I was eating right. I did not realize that unless bread is labeled as "100%" whole wheat, it usually only contains about 30% whole wheat flour, therefore 70% of the bread is processed white flour. I really believed that having tomato and lettuce (iceberg lettuce which has virtually no nutritive value) on a cheeseburger was the same as having a couple of servings of broccoli. I believed that an order of french fries was the same as having a serving of carrots. I actually thought that a box of chocolate covered cherries was healthy. Okay, not really. Most importantly, I did not have any idea just how harmful sugar is to the human body. I did not smoke or do drugs. I drank alcoholic beverages in moderation, but not on a daily basis or in large amounts. Overall, I considered myself a reasonably healthy person. I was not sickly nor on any medications, so I believed I was in very good health and that I was the last person who would ever get cancer.

We were cruising along like a typical American family: Linda and I each working a full-time job, raising a 15 month-old son, and going to church. The date was May 8th in the year 2000. It was a typical spring day in Jacksonville, FL. The weather was hot, humid, and sunny. I woke up that morning feeling miserable. I had a high fever and ached all over. For all I knew, I had the flu. I assumed it was just the flu and I was just going to let it runs its course, but when the symptoms did not improve after several days (not to mention the yellow-green color that I was turning), I decided I needed to go to the doctor. Linda knew I was really sick when I was willing to go to the doctor. I was never the type to go to the doctor for every little sniffle. I only went when I was really, really sick. If I got a cold or bronchitis, I would let it run its course, only relenting if I ran a high fever I could not shake.

Cancer, the Most Feared Word in the English Language

After several questions and tests, the doctor decided I needed to have my gall bladder checked. I was admitted to the hospital immediately with the intention that my gall bladder would be removed. Linda and Daniel spent the night in the hospital with me. However, after a few more tests, it was determined that I had hepatitis, not a bad gall bladder. The gall bladder surgery was cancelled, and after a week and more tests, it was determined that I had Epstein Barr Virus, which was affecting my liver (causing the hepatitis symptoms, mostly jaundice), which it does in about 20% of cases. (I think they got the idea for the TV show House from my case. Unfortunately, I have not received any royalty checks…yet. I am still holding my breath.) Therefore, I was sent home to rest and recuperate, as there is no cure and really no treatment for Epstein Barr Virus.

I was told I might be on bed rest for months. To be honest, I was kind of looking forward to being on forced bed rest for a while. Since our son was born 15 months prior, I was feeling worn out (probably a factor in getting sick). At the time Linda got pregnant, she had a job as a schoolteacher and I was a field estimator for a construction specialties company. We could not survive on one salary, and we had no family close by to watch our son after he was born. Since having a stranger watch our newborn child every day was never an option for us, we had to come up with an alternative solution. Our salaries were about the same, and since it would be easier for me to make money doing home improvement and handyman jobs on afternoons and weekends, we decided that Linda would continue to teach and I would start a handyman business. Linda would go to work (as a schoolteacher) during the day and I would keep Daniel. Then when Linda got home, I would go out and work on odd jobs (handyman stuff, remodeling jobs, etc.). I would work every afternoon and evening, and every Saturday. Also, I would get up during the night with our son since Linda had to get up early and go to work. The idea was that I could nap during the day to make up for getting up during the night; things did not quite work out that way, since I am not a big napper. I would only get 5 or 6 hours of sleep at night, and then stay up all day, and work into the evening. I was constantly tired as a result of this schedule. I am sure this was one of several contributing factors in my illness. Mothers will always tell you "sleep, sleep, sleep, when the baby sleeps". There is a reason for this. To summarize, the thought of not having to work for a few months was a welcome change to me. Little did I know the next 8 months would be anything but a respite.

My mother came and stayed with us and helped out so Linda could continue working. Less than two weeks into my "sabbatical", I had an episode. One evening I became very short of breath; I felt like I could not breathe, like I was going to suffocate. This passed, I felt normal again, and I went on to bed. Early the next morning, I woke up short of breath again. After a few moments, it passed again. I did not feel compelled to go to the emergency room (as it was before office hours for my doctor), but once my doctor was in, and considering the fact that I was *blue*, my mom sent us to the doctor. Linda called the doctor and told them what had happened; they said to come in right away.

The receptionist took one look at me and rushed me into an exam room. The doctor checked me over and ordered an x-ray. The x-ray indicated severe congestion in both lungs. The doctor diagnosed double pneumonia (which was appropriate based on the information at the time) and had me admitted to the hospital for treatment. After 3 or 4 days of treatment for pneumonia, I was not getting any better. It was obvious to the doctors that I did not have pneumonia; what was not obvious was what was wrong. There were only two ways to determine what was going on in there: a bronchoscopy or an open-lung biopsy.

A bronchoscopy is a procedure that allows your doctor to look at your airway through a thin viewing instrument called a bronchoscope. The throat is numbed to prevent the gag reflex, and a thin viewing instrument is inserted, down through the throat, and into the lungs. During a bronchoscopy, your doctor will examine your throat, larynx, trachea, and lower airways. A bronchoscopy is used for many different reasons; in my case it was used to attempt to take a sample of my lung to examine.

A lung biopsy removes a small piece of lung tissue, which can be looked at under a microscope. The open lung biopsy, one of four lung biopsy methods, was used on me. An open lung biopsy uses surgery to make a cut (incision) between the ribs and remove a sample of lung tissue. An open biopsy is usually done when the other methods of lung biopsy have not been successful, cannot be used, or when a larger piece of lung tissue is needed for a diagnosis.

Obviously, even though the bronchoscopy is hit or miss, since it is much less intrusive (than the open-lung biopsy) it is generally tried first. A bronchoscopy is not a lot of fun, but as I would find out, it is a walk in the park compared to an open-lung biopsy. The bronchoscopy was performed, but it did not yield any information, so I was scheduled for an open-lung biopsy. It is basically an operation. You are put under general anesthetic and you are cut open so they can take a piece of your lung for tests. Everything went smoothly, and we were told that they had to send the sample off to Syracuse (NY) to find out what I had. We would find out later that our doctors in Jacksonville thought it was cancer, but they wanted to get confirmation (second opinion) before telling me that I had cancer.

While I say everything went smoothly, that is not to say it was like having your teeth cleaned. In order to drain the fluids in your chest cavity that result from the procedure, a chest tube is inserted that is attached to a large plastic container that collects the fluid. This tube is as big around as a man's finger. The tube stays in for a couple of days or so. As you might imagine, between the suction effect and the process of your skin starting to attach to the tube, removing the chest tube is neither easy nor painless. When the young man (who was to remove my chest tube) began explaining to me the removal process, I asked him if it would hurt. He was refreshingly honest. Many times, doctors or nurses will downplay the pain or discomfort of a procedure (I wish they would just be honest and say, "This is going to hurt you more than it is going to hurt me."). He said, "I will not lie to you, it is tremendously painful. But it will be quick". He said it had been described to him as feeling like getting hit in the side with a baseball bat. I would liken it to getting shot. Although I have never been shot, I imagine that I now know how it feels. It was quick though. So I now had this six inch long curved scar (where they made the incision to get into my lung), with what looks like a bullet hole scar just below it. After the second open lung biopsy I would have months later, on the other lung, I had a long scar on each side of my chest, and a scar that looked like a bullet hole just below. I like to jokingly tell how I got the scars fighting off a gang with guns and knives.

Cancer, the Most Feared Word in the English Language

When he received confirmation from the lab in Syracuse, my doctor met with me and Linda, and gave us the diagnosis: "Cancer, you have cancer."

Cancer, the most feared word in the English language. Despite the advances in medical technology and treatment, many, many people still die from cancer. In the year 2000 (the year I was diagnosed) approximately 1.2 million people were diagnosed with cancer (approximately 550,000 people died from cancer.) In 2008 approximately 1.4 million people were diagnosed with cancer, and approximately 565,000 people died from cancer. (Footnote_1)

I was told I had non-Hodgkin's Lymphoma. The doctor said that, although there are no guarantees, it was a very treatable type of cancer. I was given some medical treatment to stabilize my condition until chemotherapy could start (several weeks later), and went home to digest this earth-shattering news.

How did I get cancer? What caused it? Was it something I could have prevented? Was it some kind of environmental factor I was exposed to? Not that knowing the cause would have changed anything, either the course of treatment or the outcome, but I think this was part of our coping mechanism; our way of releasing some of the stress of this unexpected blow. We scoured the internet for information on the type of cancer I had, as well as information on what might possibly have caused this. I thought about all of my experiences and all the different influences in my life and what might have caused me to get cancer.

In the Air Force, I worked as an air traffic controller in the tower. The large weather radar dome, which was mounted atop a tower, was just a few hundred yards from the control tower. We used to sit there in the control tower and joke about the weather radar tower and how it was rendering us impotent or possibly giving us cancer. In fact, I found out through a friend that one of my female coworkers (in the control tower) died from cancer a few years prior. While it was intriguing (and sad) to find out that information, it does not constitute proof that a weather radar caused my cancer. Two people out of 30 do not constitute a "cluster". If the radar dome causes cancer, it seems there would be a large number of people who worked at that base getting cancer.

As I allude to in the next chapter (I Will Never Leave You Nor Forsake You), I was subjected to many different particulates and fumes in the course of the handyman jobs I undertook. I wondered if this caused the cancer in my lungs (as I was not a smoker.) There was, of course, no way to know for certain if these things caused the cancer, but it seems logical that these factors at least contributed to my condition.

What about intangibles that we can't see or touch? Studies done over the past 30 years that examined the relationship between psychological factors, including stress, and cancer risk have produced conflicting results. Although the results of some studies have indicated a link between various psychological factors and an increased risk of developing cancer, a direct cause-and-effect relationship has not been proven.

While the direct cause and effect has not been proven, some studies indicate a there is a link between psychological factors, such as stress, and an increased risk of cancer. While I was going through treatment, I underwent some intense counseling over emotional and psychological issues from my past. I realized that I was holding unforgiveness against some people who, I feel, had

Cancer, the Most Feared Word in the English Language

hurt me or disappointed me. I methodically listed all the people who I could think of that might fit this category. I then went through and prayerfully forgave them and let go of the unforgiveness. Unforgiveness is a funny thing, it does not hurt the person who committed the wrong, but it shackles the one who refuses to forgive. We think that by holding a grudge against them, we are getting back at them, hurting them. In reality, holding unforgiveness eats away at us, holding us back, making us miserable, and making us sick. God even tells us in the Bible that if we do not forgive those who sin against us, God will not forgive our sins. Part of the Lord's Prayer leads us to practice this daily:

Forgive us our trespasses,

As we forgive those who trespass against us.

You may be wondering why I am discussing forgiveness; what does this have to do with cancer and illness. I believe, as I discuss in the chapter, "An All-Encompassing Approach," fighting a disease like cancer requires all of the weapons in our arsenal. One of the reasons so many of us are sick, despite all of the incredible advances in medicine, is that we rely on medicine, and medicine alone, in fighting disease. We would rather smoke, eat junk, and abuse our bodies, and then take a pill or have an operation. We would do better to make good choices in the first place. We would do well to return to Hippocrates' approach: rest, fresh air, a good diet, and cleanliness (augmented by medicines that are helpful).

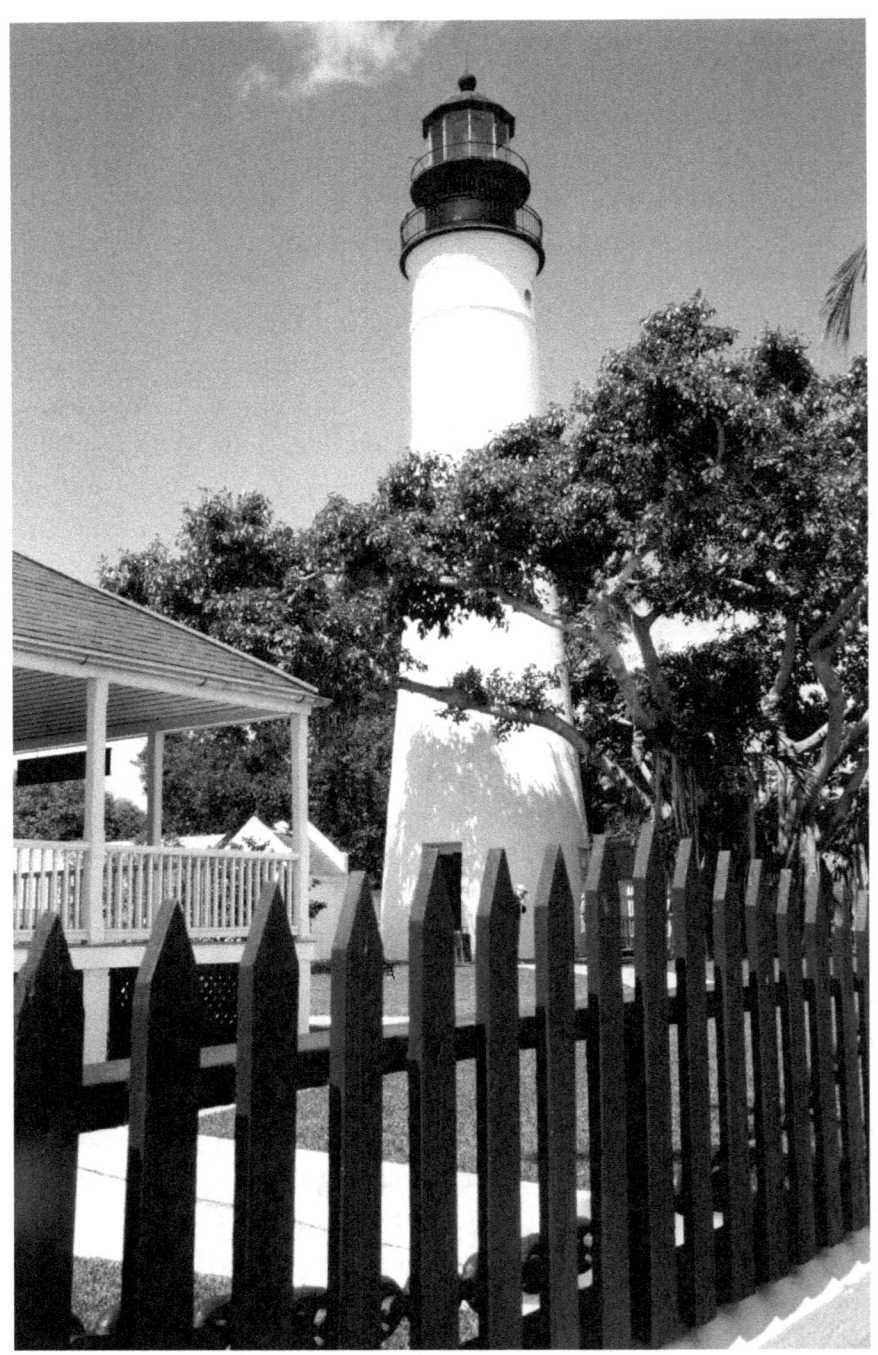

Chapter 6

I Will Never Leave You Nor Forsake You

I would like to address my thoughts and emotions at the time I found out I had cancer, as it involves my faith, which is central to this whole story. I had just been told I had cancer. This came as a total shock. When I was in the hospital, awaiting the results of the open lung biopsy, trying to figure out what it could be that I had (the doctors had told us that I had a serious lung disease, but they did not believe it was cancer), cancer was the last thing I ever expected. I could not have cancer; I was too young and healthy (or

God Said Not Yet!

so I thought).

Flash back to October 1990:

> John 3:16, 17
>
> For God so loved the world that He gave His only begotten Son,
>
> that whoever believes in Him should not perish but have everlasting life.
>
> For God did not send His Son into the world to condemn the world,
>
> but that the world through Him might be saved.

That is the Christian faith in a nutshell. Because of that assurance, God brought to my remembrance the fact that I was eternally secure through my faith in Jesus; therefore, even if this cancer led to my death, I had nothing to fear because I would be with Him in eternity. This assurance gave me great peace and an absence of fear from the beginning (in this battle with cancer). I share this because I believe that dealing with a disease like cancer takes every tool at one's disposal (spiritual, medical, dietary, emotional, etc.). I already had the foundational weapon in this battle, which was peace in my soul.

We saw many miracles from God during this time of travail. The first miracle that we saw in our lives was a financial miracle. Like most people in our culture, we were living from paycheck to paycheck, relying on both (mine and Linda's) paychecks to make ends meet. From the day I first got sick, I was unable to work (and was unable to start back to work for two years, from May 2000 until May 2002). At the time I got sick, I owned my own handyman business. This kind of work required me to perform a great variety of tasks that involved sheet rock dust, brick dust, paint fumes, gas fumes….all irritants to even the healthiest of lungs. For one job, I had to cut a doorway in a cinder block wall. On another job, I had to cut a doorway in a brick wall. These jobs required the use of a hand-held, gas-powered brick/masonry saw. Using this large, unwieldy saw was like picking up a lawn mower by the handle and using it to cut grass growing on a wall. I do not know why anyone would have grass growing on a wall, but that is the best analogy I can think of to illustrate the cumbersome nature of the saw. Even though I used a respirator mask, it did not keep out all of the dust and fumes that were generated. Many jobs required cutting pressure treated wood (which contains arsenic), sanding sheet rock compound, and breathing paint fumes. Whether or not any of these factors contributed to or caused my illness, I do not know, but I certainly was not going to take the chance of exacerbating my condition, so I did not work while going through treatment.

When we found out I had cancer, Linda communicated with our family and friends our situation. She would update everyone periodically on my condition, and everyone knew I was unable to work, however, we did not ask anyone for money nor did we tell anyone that we needed money to pay the bills. In the beginning, Linda continued working full-time. There would be times later on in this journey that Linda would be unable to work due to my worsening condition (and the fact that we had a one-year-old at home). During the whole time that I was going through medical treatment, God provided, through loving friends and family, for all our needs. Through numerous checks sent by family and friends each month, varying in amounts from $25 to $1000 (as each one was able, and moved by God), we had enough money every month to meet all our needs. The total amount was always generally the same amount; just what we needed, no more and no less. This was a demonstration of God's love for us, and our family and friends' love and generosity for which we will always be grateful (as well as their obedience to God, as we believe that God laid it on their hearts to help provide for our needs).

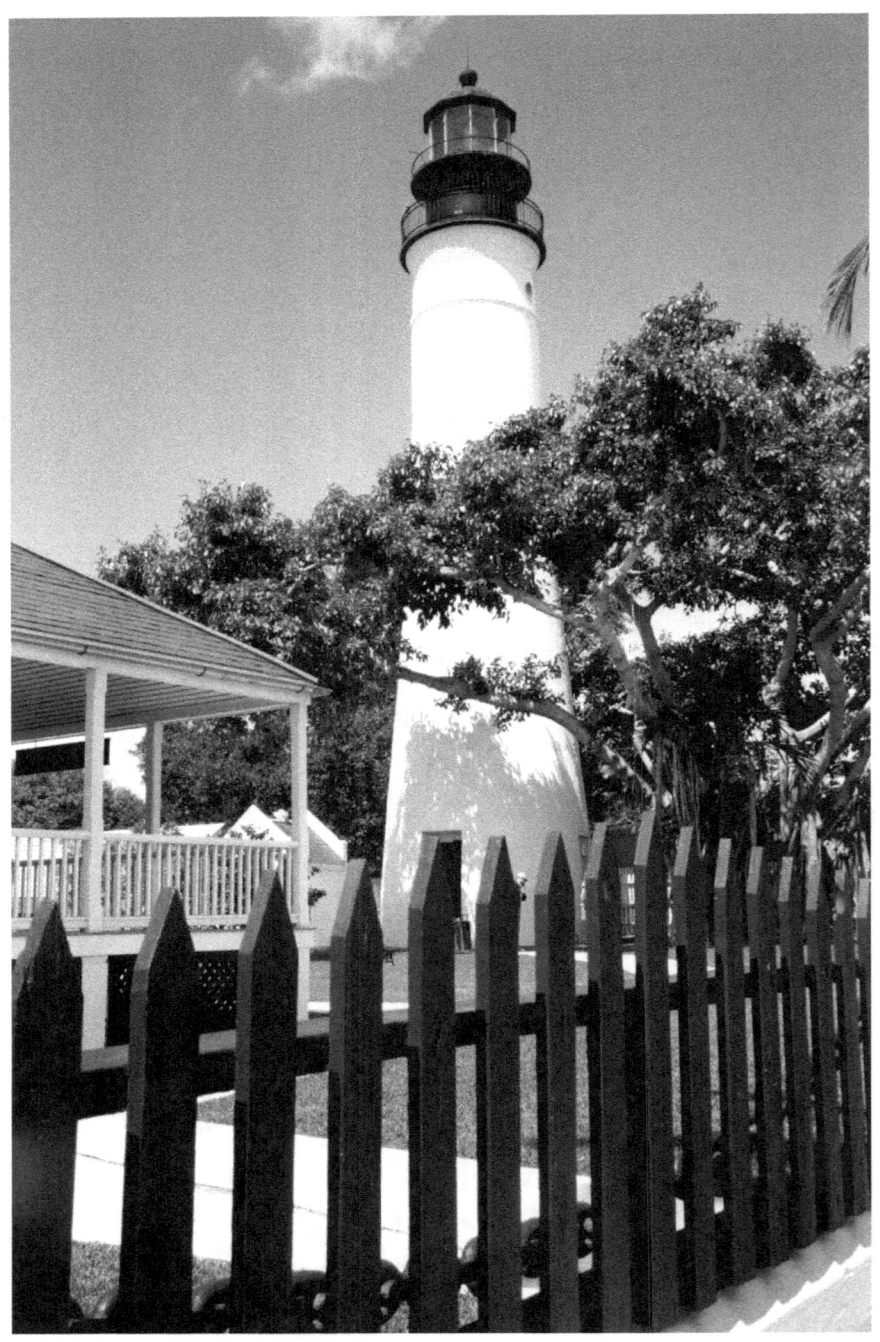

Chapter 7

Chemotherapy and Other Adventures

A bone marrow biopsy was performed to determine if the cancer had spread to my bone marrow. Most patients have this test done by a hematologist in a clinic procedure area. You wear a hospital gown during the procedure. A sedative may be injected at this time. (If you are prescribed a sedative in pill form, you will be instructed to take it ahead of time.)

Most patients have bone marrow sampled from the pelvis. You lie on your stomach and the doctor feels the bones at the top of your buttock. An area on your buttock is cleaned with soap. A local anesthetic is injected to numb the skin and the tissue underneath the skin in the sampling area. This causes some very brief stinging.

A small cut is made in the skin to allow the biopsy needle to be placed through the skin. This needle is about half as wide as a pencil and has a handle on one end that your doctor holds while he or she moves it through your bone. The biopsy needle is moved through the bone with a twisting motion, as a corkscrew would be moved through a cork. When the needle has passed through the top layer of bone, your doctor uses a syringe to pull a liquid sample of your bone marrow cells through the needle. For most patients, the suction used in this liquid collection causes a pain in the buttock for a few seconds; this is why pain medicine is usually given in preparation for the biopsy. (Footnote_2)

After taking the liquid sample, the doctor carefully moves the needle a little bit further into the bone marrow to collect a second sample of marrow called a core biopsy. This core biopsy is a small solid piece of bone marrow, with not just the liquid and cells but also the fat and bone fibers that hold them together. After the needle is pulled out, this solid sample can be pushed out of the needle with a wire so that it can be examined under a microscope. Pressure is applied to your buttock at the biopsy location for a few minutes, until you are not at risk of bleeding. A bandage is placed on your buttock. Thankfully, the test came back negative.

The chemotherapy treatments started in late June 2000. The actual treatments were (reasonably) benign. Other than the needle prick to start the IV lead, there was no pain to speak of. As a matter of fact, I was given Benadryl (to prevent the nausea caused by chemotherapy), and usually slept for most of the treatment (which would last 3-4 hours). So, other than the trouble of getting out and going to the oncologist's office, the chemotherapy treatments were not all that bad.

The side effects were another matter (although I would find out later, when my dosage was increased dramatically, the side effects I experienced in the first few months of treatment were minimal). I felt nauseous for a few days (but it was mild, and there was no vomiting), and my sense of taste was affected. Foods did not taste bad necessarily, just different (it was great, I could eat a peanut butter and jelly sandwich, and it tasted like lobster! We saved a lot of money on food while I was sick.) Most foods did not taste like they normally did.

My energy was diminished somewhat, but nothing like I would experience after my last few chemotherapy treatments. I would feel weak and tired for a few days, kind of like the way one feels when sick with the flu: generally run down. Constipation was also a problem.

While the first few months of chemotherapy passed by without incident, I did experience complications in September. I caught some kind of infection in my lungs and had to be hospitalized. I was on a variety of antibiotics, via an IV drip, around the clock, for one solid week. One bag would finish, and the nurse would take it down and hang another bag. At the end of the week, I had a reaction to the antibiotics and experienced extreme shortness of breath (similar to the episodes I had when I first got sick. It was terrible; I literally felt like I was suffocating. Finally, I was given a shot to counteract the shortness of breath (perhaps steroids, I do not remember for certain), and I survived the first of many tribulations: incidents in which the cancer tried to take me, but God said, "Not Yet!" I recovered from that episode, and felt relatively good for the next couple of months (until Thanksgiving weekend). I got back to the business of receiving treatment once a week, having blood work done once a week, and lying around, resting and waiting.

During the course of my treatment, I had to go once a week, on Friday, for chemotherapy or an experimental alternative drug. I received chemotherapy once every three weeks, and on the two Fridays in between, I was treated with Rituxan. Once a week, usually at the beginning of the week, I had to have my blood drawn so my doctor could monitor my blood work. During each of my several stays in the hospital, I was stuck at least once every day for blood work. (This always occurred at around five o'clock in the morning. Do these people not realize that when you are sick you need your rest? Why do they have to wake you up in the middle of a deep sleep and stick a needle in your arm?) Needles do not bother me (I do not get terrified and sweaty and pass out when I see a needle), but the little prick does not feel good either. Early on, it was not too bad to get stuck twice a week, but that would change. One thing chemotherapy does to your body is that it causes your veins to become hard and brittle. When your veins become hard and brittle, it becomes increasingly more difficult for a lab tech or nurse to find a vein from which to draw blood. Sometimes the vein will "blow out" when the needle hits it, and other times the needle will simply glance off the vein. After a month or so, it got to the point where the nurse or lab tech would have to stick me two or three times (occasionally even four or five times) to get into a vein (sometimes having to switch arms). After a while, I started dreading getting blood work or an IV.

Chemotherapy and Other Adventures

The oxygen level of my blood had to be monitored constantly, as the cancer was affecting my lungs. The oxygen level of the blood is measured in percentage, with optimal level being 100%. When I was doing reasonably well during treatment, my blood oxygen level was 96%; there were times when my blood oxygen level dropped to 90%. While 90% sounds like plenty of oxygen, it was a great concern when my level dropped to 90%. One way to measure a person's blood oxygen level is a little device that clips on to the end of the finger. This device reads a person's pulse and blood oxygen level. Although this sounds like something Dr. McCoy would use (Star Trek reference. No, I am not a Trekkie, if I were a Trekkie, I would not explain the reference, I would just assume everyone knew what I was referring to), we are not quite there yet (technologically speaking). This device is not extremely accurate. In order to get an accurate blood oxygen level reading, your blood had to be tested. However, the blood in your veins cannot be used, as it has been used by your cells and is returning for replenishment. The purpose of testing your blood oxygen level is to determine how efficiently your blood is being oxygenated (an indication of how well your lungs are functioning. Therefore, blood had to be drawn from an artery. The artery of choice for this particular procedure was the artery in your wrist. The nurse who performed this procedure explained to me, that because of the location of the artery (deep in the wrist close to the bone), it would be extremely painful (much worse than getting stuck for blood work). Since doctors and nurses usually down play pain to patients, I was expecting the most painful experience of my life. Getting a needle stuck into your wrist, right up to the bone. Sounds painful, does it not? I readied myself, grabbing the armrest of my chair tightly, expecting to go through the ceiling when she inserted the needle. She stuck the needle in my wrist, drew out some blood, and removed the needle. I could not believe it; there was almost no pain. I was expecting unimaginable pain, yet it was less of a prick than I felt getting my blood drawn. I do not know if my senses were dulled from all the chemotherapy or if God prevented the needle from hitting any nerves, but I was very grateful to be spared the pain. Maybe it was a case of mind over matter. If it was, I do not know how I did it nor can I replicate the process when I need it.

While I had many interesting and painful experiences through my first six months of treatment, the most dramatic was yet to come.

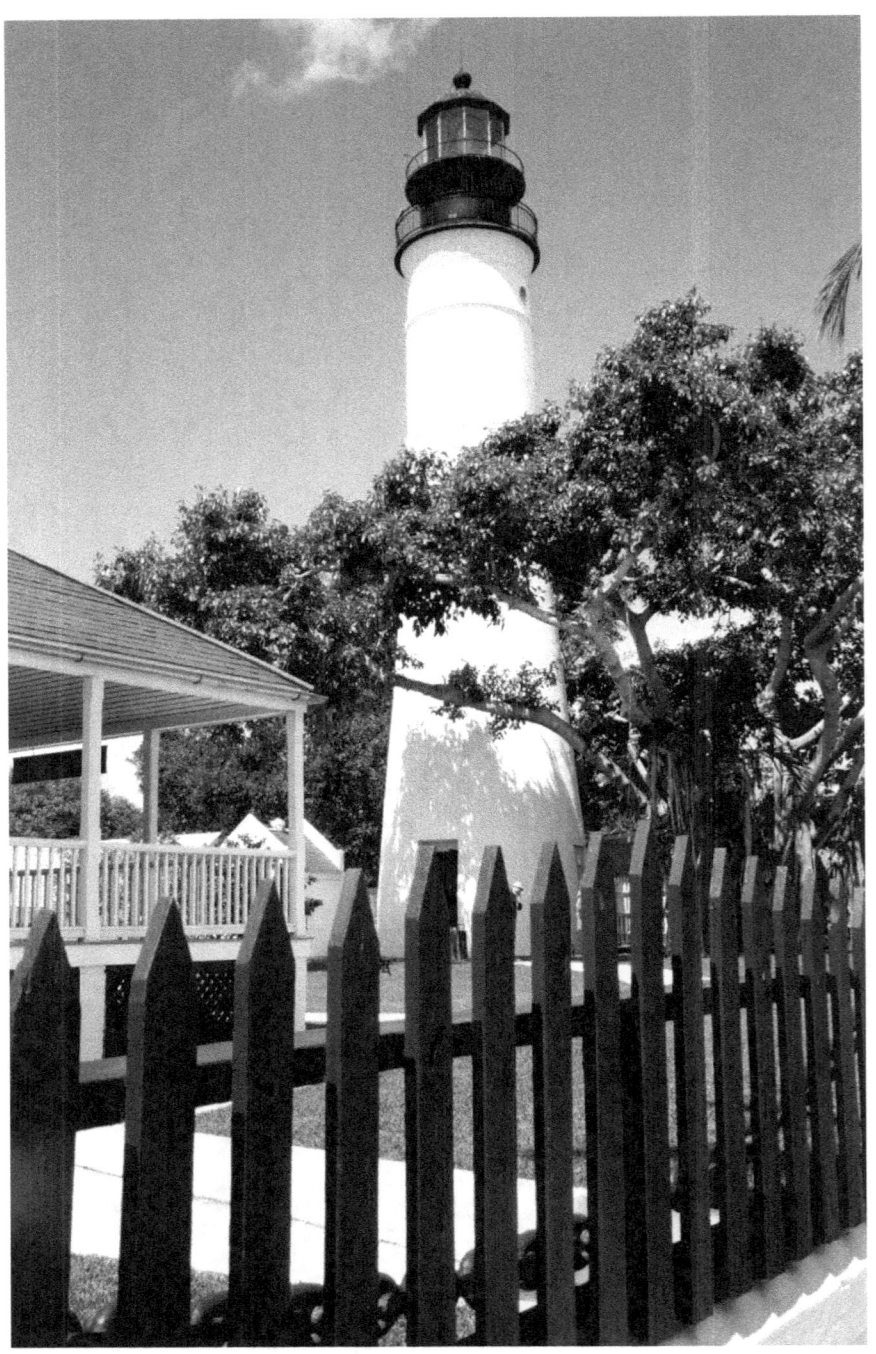

Chapter 8

Not Exactly the Most Wonderful Time of the Year

Five months into my treatments (mid-November), I was doing reasonably well (or so I thought); I was not in remission, but I seemed to be doing okay. For Thanksgiving, our friends, Rick and Lori, had us over to their house for dinner. Daniel, Linda and I, Rick and Lori, their two daughters and Lori's parents, made for a full house. A beautifully decorated house and turkey and all the trimmings set the stage for a traditional Thanksgiving dinner. I was feeling good and enjoyed the company of good friends and a delicious Thanksgiving dinner.

As Thanksgiving weekend came to a close, I started going downhill fast. I was admitted to the hospital immediately. X-rays and a CT scan indicated that there were significant obstructions in my lungs. While the x-rays and scan showed obstructions, there was no way to know for certain what was causing the obstructions. Most likely, it was still the cancer, but it could be pneumonia, other infections, or scar tissue. The only way to find out for sure was the good old open-lung biopsy. My lungs were in worse shape than when I had the first open-lung biopsy, significantly worse, and things did not go smoothly this time. I stopped breathing in the middle of the procedure and had to be revived on the table. After being revived, I was awake (without any anaesthetic) briefly until they were sure I was stable. It was the most painful, horrifying experience I have ever been through.

While it was a very harrowing experience, I did make it through. The cancer tried to take me, but God said, "Not yet!" The result of the biopsy was cancer; and it was worse than when I started chemotherapy. Five months of treatment and I was worse, not better. Obviously, the treatments I was getting were not doing the job. This news was, to say the least, discouraging. The next step was to try a stronger dose of chemotherapy (the thinking being that the previous doses were too weak. In addition, this was to determine if I would be a candidate for the bone marrow transplant procedure. Essentially, we were told, if the cancer did not respond to a stronger dose of chemotherapy, I would not be a candidate for the bone marrow transplant procedure, which would mean that all hope was lost, at least as far as medical

Not Exactly the Most Wonderful Time of the Year

treatment is concerned. I would discover that as long as God is involved, there is always hope.)

During the previous five months I had not lost my hair nor felt especially incapacitated. There would be a few days of weakness and constipation following each chemotherapy treatment, but nothing major. I remember thinking, during the first few months of treatment, that everything I had heard (about going through chemotherapy) was blown out of proportion (or medical advances had dramatically reduced the side effects). During this run of stronger treatments, I began to get a taste of what I was expecting when I started this journey. I lost all of my hair (I do mean ALL of my hair, as in ALL of my hair; I did not even have any eyebrows). I could barely get off the couch (to go to the bathroom) for about a week. I did not feel much like eating. It was rough. Think of the flu doubled or tripled.

It was now December of 2000. While everyone else was doing their Christmas shopping and planning parties, I was fighting for my life. That December was a long month. As near as I can remember, I spent 21 of the 31 days that December in the hospital. I started the month in the hospital, got to go home for about a week, then had to check back in due to complications. When Christmas Eve came, even though I was not doing very well, I was able to talk my doctor into letting me go home for a day or two for Christmas. Linda's parents had come to town to spend Christmas with us, but I asked them to leave so Linda, Daniel and I could be alone. We thought this might be my last Christmas, and we wanted to be alone as a family. Her parents respectfully obliged. I checked out of the hospital around noon on Christmas Eve, and then had to be back first thing in the morning, the day after

God Said Not Yet!

Christmas. Christmas that year was not extremely festive, but it was a very special time. It was just Linda, Daniel (22 months old) and me, and our Golden Retriever Dusty (the best dog ever). We opened presents, had a nice little meal, watched "It's a Wonderful Life" and counted our blessings. We got to spend Christmas together and at home (not in a hospital room), I was still alive, and we had each other.

At this point, things did not look good for me. It looked like this would be my last Christmas. While I was not afraid die, the thought of my demise caused me great heartache, not out of fear, but out of concern for my son Daniel and my wife Linda. I did not want to leave them alone in this world. I remember the words I prayed to God. I said, "Lord, my life is yours, and it is up to you when my life is over. I am not afraid to die and I yield to your will, and if it is my time to go, take me. However, I do not want to die. I do not want my son to grow up without his daddy. I want to be around to watch him grow up." I also thought about the fact that if I died my son would never know me as his father. I do not remember anything prior to the age of six or so, and Daniel was not yet two years old at that point. I knew that if I died, he would soon forget me, and in his memory, it would be as if I never existed. Selfishly, I wanted to live so my son would know that I was his father. Only God knows if I was destined to live on or if that prayer changed things, but the point is I was wholeheartedly submitted to God's will, whatever it might be.

While I was in the hospital that December, an older (Episcopal) priest, and his wife, from our church came to visit me. Bob and Ann were the sweetest little couple you could imagine. They loved the Lord and would do anything for anyone. Father

Not Exactly the Most Wonderful Time of the Year

Bob and Ann visited with me for a while, prayed over me, and read an excerpt from the Bible to me. The passage, which Fr. Bob read to me from the Old Testament, would serve two purposes: renewing God's call in my life and serving as an anchor through times in the months ahead when all seemed hopeless:

Isaiah 61:1-3

The Spirit of the Lord GOD *is* upon Me,
Because the LORD has anointed Me
To preach good tidings to the poor;
He has sent Me to heal the brokenhearted,
To proclaim liberty to the captives,
And the opening of the prison to *those who are* bound;
To proclaim the acceptable year of the LORD,
And the day of vengeance of our God;
To comfort all who mourn,

To console those who mourn in Zion,
To give them beauty for ashes,
The oil of joy for mourning,
The garment of praise for the spirit of heaviness;
That they may be called trees of righteousness,
The planting of the LORD, that He may be glorified.

As Father Bob began reading that passage of scripture to me, I was overcome with emotion. It resonated in my spirit that God was reestablishing His calling on me to work with teenagers, specifically those who need another chance and need direction in their life (termed as "at-risk", "troubled", etc.). From the phrase,

God Said Not Yet!

"He has sent me to heal the brokenhearted," to giving them "The garment of praise for the spirit of heaviness," I knew that God was telling me it was time to get back to working with hurting youth. This buoyed my spirits through some difficult times ahead (over the following month or two). When it looked like I was going to die, the memory of that moment (when God confirmed His call on me) carried me through; I knew I was not going to die even though things looked that way.

Back in the summer, when I was diagnosed with cancer and began chemotherapy treatments, I had put my dream of pursuing a career in architecture on hold. I contacted the staff at the University of Cincinnati and informed them that I would not be there in the fall and why. Graciously, they offered their prayers and well-wishes. I guess I thought that once I was well, I would resume my pursuit of this dream. With this renewal of God's call on my life to work with troubled youth, I knew it was time to let go of my dream once and for all. This dream, which had bubbled up within me several times in my life, only to be beaten back down by self doubt; the dream which I had finally stepped out aggressively to pursue, would have to be put to rest, given over to God. Perhaps I will get to be an architect in heaven.

After going through several chemotherapy treatments of increased intensity, tests revealed that the cancer seemed to retreat a little, not enough to suggest continuing this course of treatment, but enough to give hope that the bone marrow transplant procedure could work. So it was determined that I was a candidate for the bone marrow transplant procedure. My doctors strongly recommended that I submit to the bone marrow transplant procedure, and an appointment was made for me at the

Not Exactly the Most Wonderful Time of the Year

University of Florida Cancer Center to meet with the doctors for a consultation.

My body was deteriorating; I had little energy left. I had no hair and I was pale and ashen; this was one of those times when it looked like the cancer was going to win. Though it seemed like I was going to die, I had to cling to the hope that God's call gave me.

We prepared to make the trip to Gainesville for the consultation. While the consultation was not exactly something fun to look forward to, getting out of the house for a road trip was exciting. Gainesville, FL is about a two hour drive from Jacksonville, FL. The drive takes you through Middleburg, Starke, Hampton and Waldo. You pass through pine forests, palmetto lined roads, quaint small towns and the alligator infested swamps of central Florida: all in all a very peaceful, relaxing drive and an enjoyable diversion. My mom and dad, who were visiting with us at the time, drove down with us. They went with us for moral support and to watch Daniel while Linda and I met with the medical team for the consultation. While the drive down was relaxing, I felt an uneasiness, a gnawing anxiety, beginning to germinate within my spirit. At the time, I thought it was just normal nerves associated with meeting new doctors about a new procedure I would have to undergo. I would soon find out there was more to it than that.

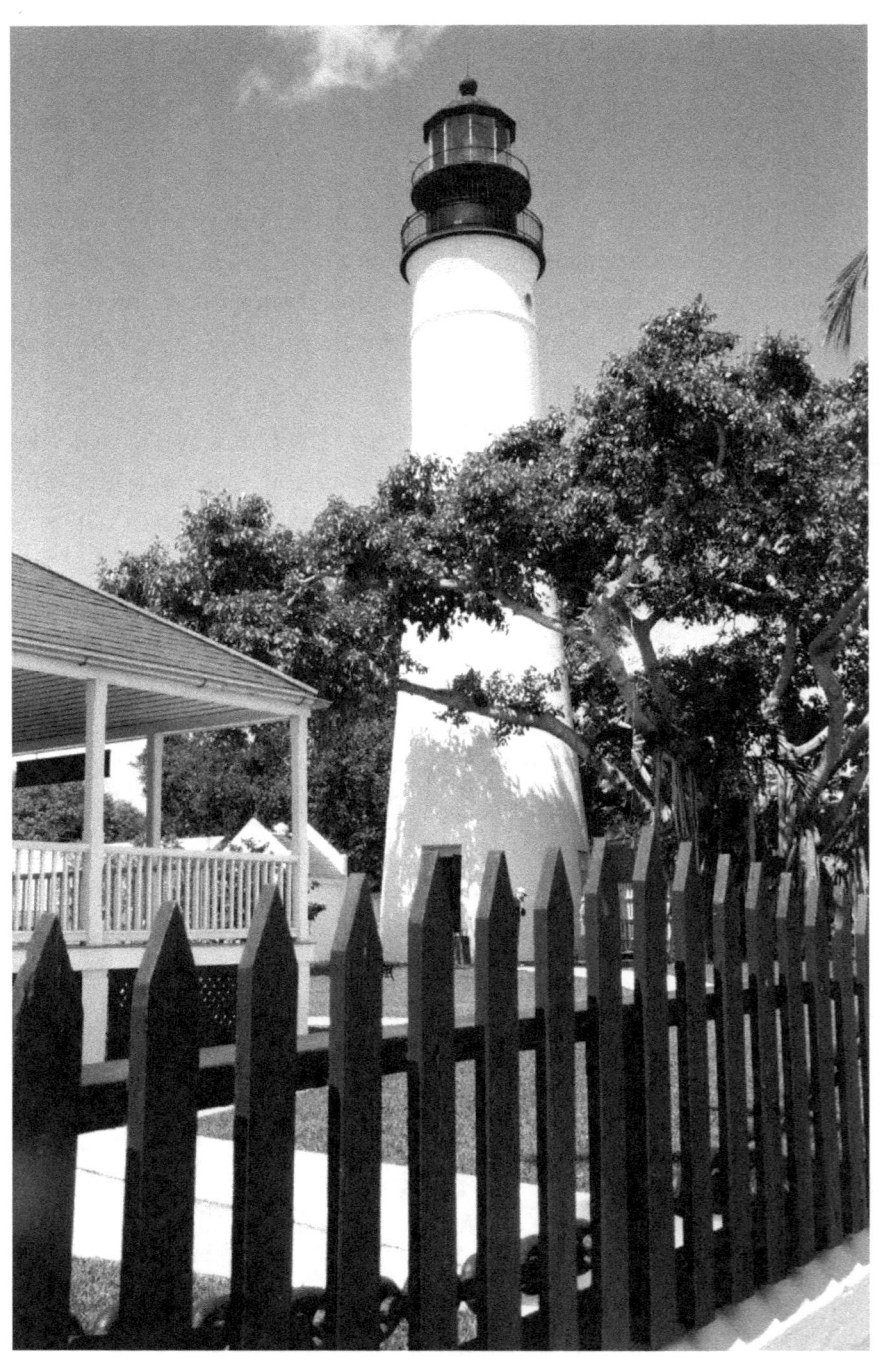

Chapter 9

This is Your Last Hope

The procedure, the Bone Marrow Transplant, is actually a chemotherapy treatment. A bone marrow transplant is a procedure where special cells (called stem cells) that are normally found in the bone marrow are taken out, filtered, and given back either to the same person or to another person. Stem cell transplants are used to restore the stem cells when the bone marrow has been destroyed by disease, chemotherapy, or radiation. Bone marrow produces stem cells. These cells eventually develop into blood cells. Bone marrow is a critical part of the body because it is the body's main blood cell "factory." If something is wrong with the marrow, a person can become very ill, even die. (Footnote 3)

After stem cells are harvested, the individual is treated with a powerful dose of chemotherapy. The healthy stem cells are then infused into the individual. With regards to the Bone Marrow Transplant Procedure, I do not remember the exact statistics, and I am sure they change from year to year, but I do remember the number was small. The percentage of people who survived the process and saw their disease go into remission was well below 50%. Not encouraging, but it was implied that this was my last, only hope.

For the first time since being diagnosed, I was feeling very distressed. I knew that this procedure, which my doctors were recommending, was pretty much a case of "we don't have anything else to try." The cancer was winning, the standard treatment was *not* working, and this Bone Marrow Transplant Procedure, which had a very low rate of success, was my last, only hope. As we checked in at the cancer center and waited for my appointment, those twinges of anxiety, that sense of dread that started on the drive down (which I had not felt before this trip), began to grow stronger. Over the next couple of days after the consultation, those twinges started building to a crescendo. For several days, I was consumed with the gnawing feeling that this procedure would be the end for me, a literal "dead-end". I could barely function. I was sinking into darkness, hopelessness, and despair. It was as if I was standing out in the cold, under a dark night sky with no stars and no moon: no light whatsoever.

This is Your Last Hope

Then, like a brilliant shooting star illuminating the dark night sky, an amazing thought overtook my emotions; for the first time during my eight month battle with cancer, I had the revelation that just because the doctors said I needed a certain treatment (the Bone Marrow Transplant Procedure), that did not mean I had to submit to the treatment; the choice was still mine. Up to this point, whatever the doctors said or recommended I followed blindly. I do not know if it was my military training kicking in, or just that I trusted the doctors implicitly, but I did not question what the doctors said, and was not hesitant about any of the procedures the doctors prescribed. After meeting with the doctors at the bone marrow transplant clinic, for the first time, I was not inclined to follow the doctors' advice. For some people in the same situation this might be the best course of action, but for me, I did not feel that it was. As a matter of fact, I was very reluctant to follow this course of treatment. I believe this was the Lord's leading, as He knows all. Jesus promised us that God the Father would send us the Holy Spirit to teach us all things:

John 14:26

But the Helper, the Holy Spirit, whom the Father will send in My name, He will teach you all things, and bring to your remembrance all things that I said to you.

John 16:13

However, when He, the Spirit of truth, has come,

He will guide you into all truth.

God Said Net Yet!

Of course, this was a very difficult decision. Basically, since the doctors were recommending this procedure that has a relatively low survival/remission rate, I knew the doctors felt this was my only hope (that I was going to die from cancer if I did not follow this course of treatment), even though, as one of my doctors put it: "Because of the condition of your lungs, there is a high probability of mortality (death)."

It seems that I was faced with two choices: submit to the bone marrow transplant and probably die, or refuse the bone marrow transplant and certainly die. Regardless of the fact that (according to the doctors) the bone marrow transplant procedure was my only chance for survival, I felt very strongly that I was not supposed to submit to this procedure. I had no indication of any other options I might have. My situation, it seemed, was hopeless.

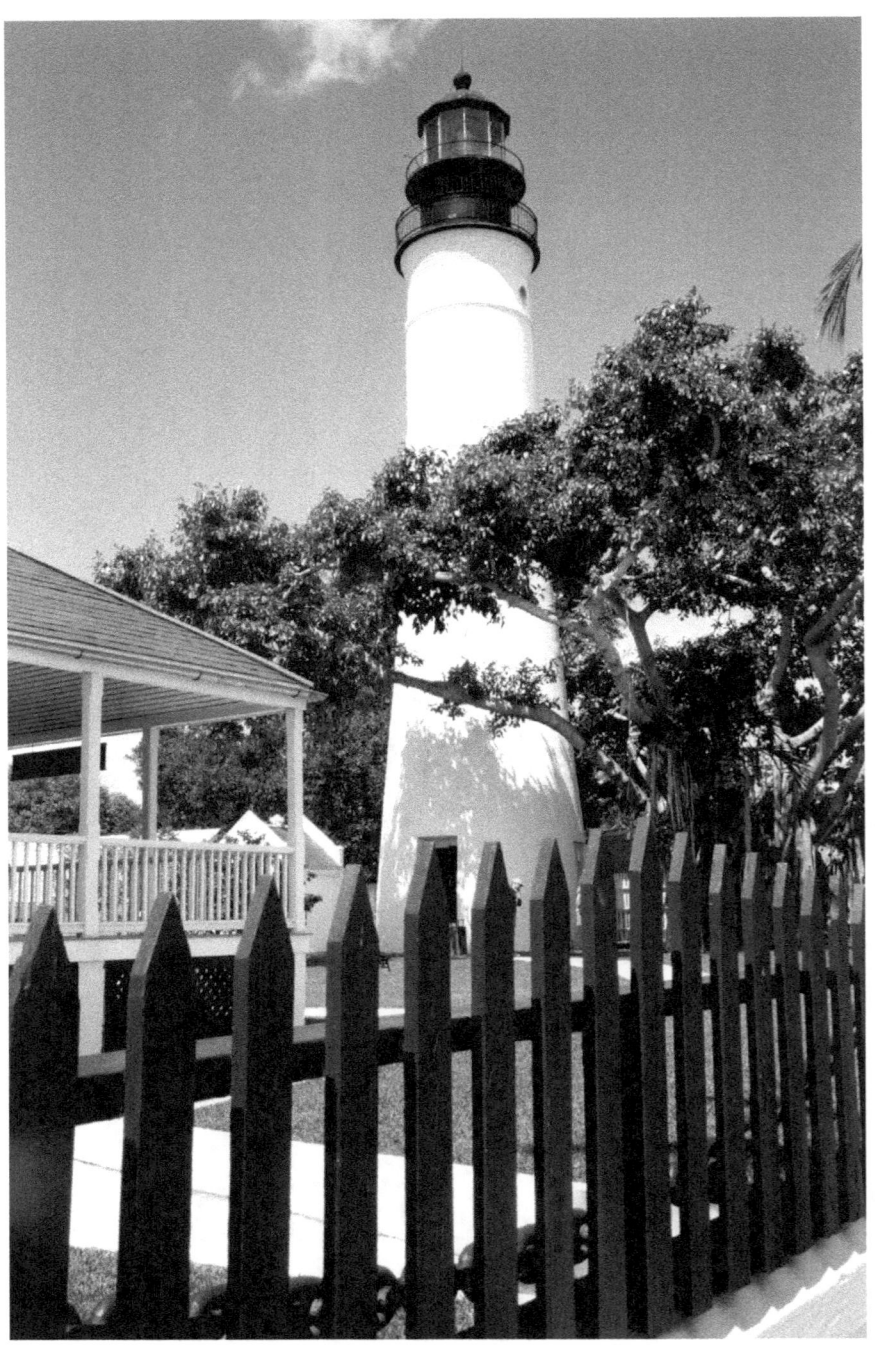

Chapter 10

The Peace of God

I was faced with a literal life-or-death decision. Continue on the present course of treatment and die from cancer. Submit to the bone marrow transplant, and probably die from complications. Walk away from medical treatment and die from cancer. I had never before been faced with such a difficult decision. I talked to a good friend of mine (Russ) for advice on how to make such a difficult decision, how to know which way to turn. I firmly believed I was not supposed to go through with the bone marrow transplant or take any more chemotherapy, but I did not know of any other options. My friend told me that when he had to make a difficult decision, he would make the decision he believed he should make. Then he would pray and ask God for confirmation, and sit on it for 24 hours. He told me that if it was the right decision, he would have peace about it, if it was the wrong decision, there would be a lack of peace, a sense of uneasiness.

Russ is a good man of God. I highly respect Russ and covet his advice. I got to know Russ just a couple of years after coming to know the Lord. I had driven to the home of a friend from church who was hosting an in-home small group meeting. As I was walking up to the front door, I ran into Russ. He introduced himself, and (seemingly) out of the blue, asked me if I wanted to join him at the prison to help with a prison ministry he presided over. Although I had never been involved in prison work or even thought about it, I promptly and enthusiastically answered yes. This was one of those moments when I knew immediately this was something God was calling me to do. Some people might think it would be scary to think about going into a prison, but when God calls you to do something, there is no fear.

I did whatever Russ needed me to do, whether it was praying for the men, carrying his guitar, or just being there. From time to time, Russ asked me to teach a lesson (or give a sermon.) Despite struggling with Chronic Fatigue for years, Russ faithfully ministered in the prison for more than 15 years. On a few occasions, when Russ was not feeling up to going, he asked me to fill in for him. I was happy to oblige. I got to lead the singing, as well as preaching. Since I lacked Russ' musical talent, I would lead a cappella singing from the hymn book. It was not the same

The Peace of God

as singing modern praise songs to the accompaniment of Russ' guitar playing, but there was a simple, authentic atmosphere of worship nonetheless. The sound of 25-30 men singing hymns a cappella in the middle of a prison is sublime.

I was counting on Russ to give me some advice I could use in making this decision, and he did not disappoint. Linda and I got on our knees and went to the Lord in prayer. We told God that we were going to inform the doctors that I would not submit to the bone marrow transplant procedure and that I would not receive any more chemotherapy. We asked God to guide us as to whether this was the right decision or not. The Bible talks about a peace which "transcends understanding"; a peace that makes no sense in light of your circumstances; a peace that cannot be explained or even understood. (Transcend: to rise above or extend notably beyond ordinary limits.)

Philippians 4:6, 7

Be anxious for nothing, but in everything

by prayer and supplication, with thanksgiving,

let your requests be made known to God;

and the peace of God, which surpasses all understanding,

will guard your hearts and minds through Christ Jesus.

Before we even finished praying, I was filled with this peace (from God), the peace that passes/transcends/defies understanding. I knew that this was the right decision, even though I did not know what we would do next, and I knew what the doctors would say (that I was going to die). To have a complete and utter peace (when you are going against the advice of the doctors and friends and family, and you do not know what you will do next) defies logic or understanding. There should be doubt and fear and trepidation, yet there was nothing but an overwhelming peace that flooded my soul. As His Word promises, "the peace of God guarded my heart and mind through Christ Jesus."

We sat on the decision for 24 hours as my friend recommended. We still had complete peace that we were making the right decision. So we went to our doctor to tell him/her (we had a team of five oncologists) of our decision. When we informed our doctor of our decision, she was of course taken aback. She told us that, while she understood this was our decision to make, and that she respected our decision, she felt that it was her professional responsibility to inform us that my life expectancy would be months, maybe weeks. God would have something to say about that: God said, "Not Yet!"

That was February of 2001. An interesting note here. We were in a situation where we had to decide whether we would trust in (or follow the advice or leading of) God or the advice of doctors. While we were praying and dealing with this decision, we tried to call a couple (who were close friends of ours) to ask them to pray for us as we sought God's guidance. We were not able to get in touch with them. Therefore, they knew nothing about this decision we were making. Shortly after we talked to the doctors and informed them of our decision, we received an email from this couple. It was one of those forwarded emails that contained some interesting facts. This was about the Bible. There are 31,174 verses in the Bible. That being an even number, there are two verses that are the very center of the Bible: Psalm 118:8 and Psalm 118:9. These two verses are very interesting in light of the decision we had to make.

Psalm 118:8-9

8 It is better to take refuge in the LORD than to trust in man.

9 It is better to take refuge in the LORD than to trust in princes.

You could argue that doctors in our society are like princes (wealthy, respected, and revered). I want to make something clear, I am NOT saying that you should never consult or trust a doctor. What I am saying is if God is telling you one thing, and the doctors tell you something that conflicts with that, it is better to trust in the Lord than to put confidence in man. At least in my experience that was the case.

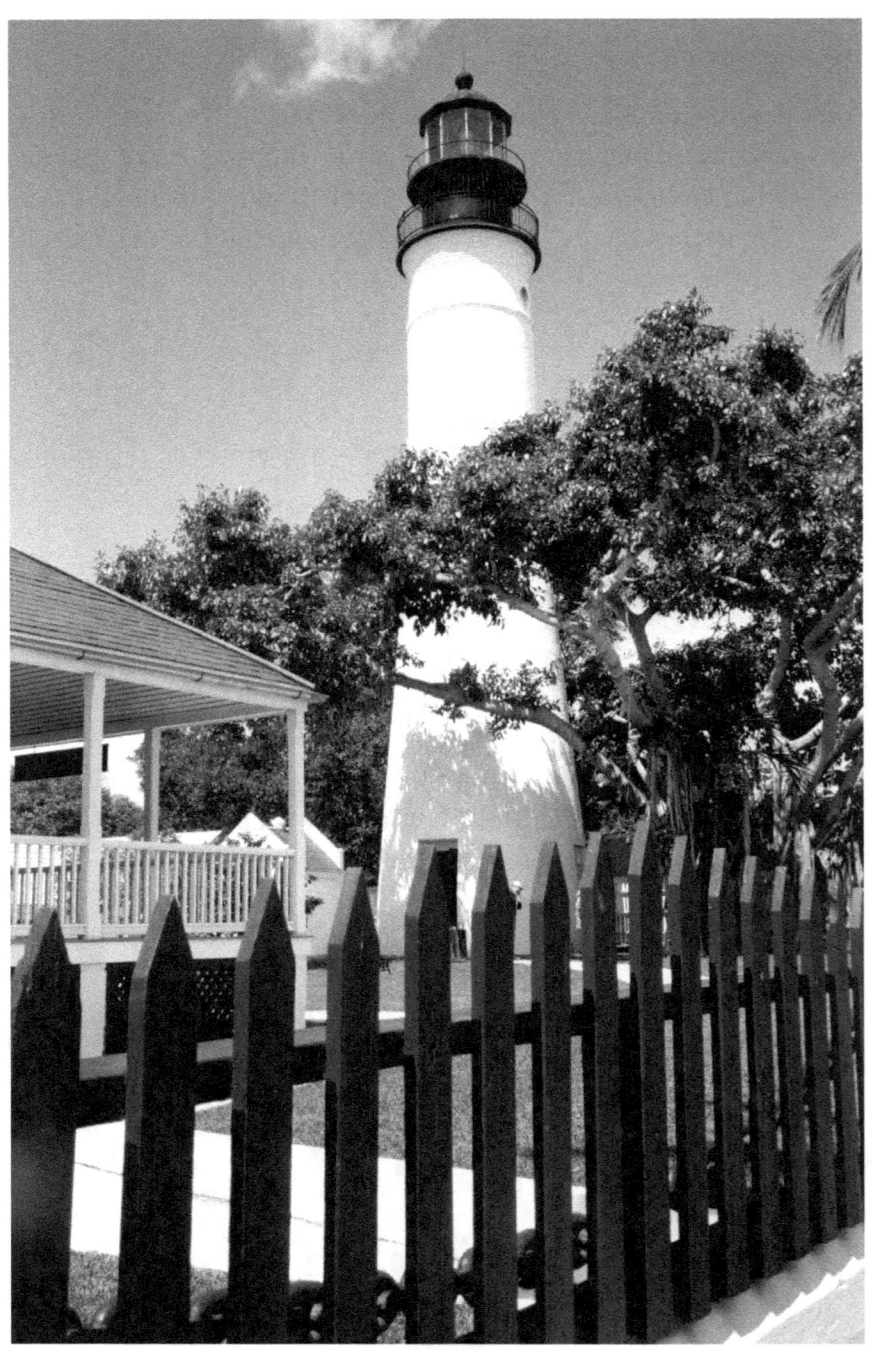

Chapter 11

A Leap of Faith

I was faced with what amounted to a leap of faith. It was as if I was standing on the edge of a cliff, and God was telling me to take a step. According to the doctors, if I walked away from medical treatment, I would surely die. God was leading me to walk away from medical treatment. If I followed God's leading, would I fall off the cliff to my death, or would His angels catch me and hold me up? I did not know what would happen, but the one thing I did know was that I was going to trust God; I was going to take the leap.

When I stepped out in faith following God's leading, I did not know what to expect next. For all I knew I was going to fall off that cliff (in other words die from the cancer). I just knew that I was supposed to refuse the bone marrow transplant procedure. Shortly after I informed my doctors of my decision to forego any further medical treatment, a friend from church gave me a book titled "Alive and Well" by Dr. Philip Binzel. After I stepped out in faith, the next section of the path was revealed.

I will elaborate on this book and the regimen I followed, but first I would like to interject some details about my thoughts and feelings, as well as my siblings and our interactions about my decision to stop all treatment.

My two sisters and my brother had been tested as possible bone marrow donors for the bone marrow transplant procedure. When we told my sisters that I was not going to do the bone marrow transplant procedure and that I was foregoing all medical treatment, they were understandably upset and concerned. They probably thought I was crazy or delirious. They did not have my individual experience with God that gave me complete peace that my life was in His hands. They, like the majority of Americans, believed that doctors have all the answers, and if a doctor says jump, you ask how high. I, too, trusted implicitly in the doctors' advice until it came to the bone marrow transplant. I knew, deep inside, that this time I was not supposed to go along with the doctor's advice. Once again, I want to stress that I am NOT recommending everyone abandon all medical advice and treatment. I am just saying that ultimately, the One who created this universe, who created you (your body), knows what is best for you. If God is leading you to take a different direction (than what the doctor says), in my opinion, it is always best to follow Him.

My sisters flew from New Jersey to Jacksonville, Florida to try to convince me to go ahead with the recommended medical treatment. I told them why I was so sure I was making the right decision, and that I would not waver. While I knew that God had plans for me and that I was going to survive, I felt I needed to try to assure my sisters. I believe that God has our life in His hands, and He knows the day and the hour that He has appointed for our life to end. I told them that maybe my time was just two or three months away, and if that were the case, God would want me to feel as good as I could and enjoy that time (I had left) with my wife, and our (almost) two year old son (as well as family and friends). If I went through with the bone marrow transplant procedure, I would have been in miserable shape for those last few months. Would it not be better to spend that final time feeling relatively good? I know that I am extremely blessed to have siblings who care so much, who were willing to be bone marrow donors, and who cared so much that they were willing to get on a plane to come see me and set me straight (as they saw it at the time). I know their intentions were good and true, and I appreciate them for that, but at the same time I knew that God wanted me to go in a different direction, and I was going to follow His lead, no matter where it led. It can be very difficult for family members to accept decisions made by their loved ones.

Now back to the book that was given to us. "Alive and Well" by Dr. Philip Binzel, chronicles Dr. Binzel's treatment of cancer patients with Laetrile. Upon reading Dr. Binzel's book, I was convinced that this treatment could be helpful for me. The alternative treatment plan involves a strict diet, vitamin and enzyme supplements, and intravenous Laetrile. I began the diet regimen right away. I will not recount the diet in detail in this book (for that I recommend you buy Dr. Binzel's book). I will just say that is a pure diet that excludes all processed food, sugar, white flour, preservatives; a diet that we would all do well to follow regardless of whether we have cancer or not. A diet, I must confess, from which I have strayed from time to time. As for the supplements and intravenous treatment, I did not start that immediately. The supplements are only necessary just prior to and during the intravenous treatments.

I have never had a problem with needles. My whole life, needles have been very easy for me. It probably has something to do with the fact that I had to get regular shots for allergies when I was young (under 10). My mother was a registered nurse so she was able to give these injections to me at home.

While needles do not bother me, I needed a break. During my eight months of chemotherapy treatments and hospitalizations, I endured many, many needle pricks. Once every week I had to get my blood drawn for tests. Once every week I had to have an IV lead (needle) put in my arm for the chemotherapy treatment. When I was hospitalized (a total of about 50 days or so over eight months) a nurse would come in every day to draw blood. In addition, after a couple months of chemotherapy treatments, your veins begin to deteriorate. They become hardened and fragile. When a needle is injected into one of your veins (whether to draw blood or to start an IV lead), the needle tends to glance off the vein or cause it to blow out. So, after the first couple of months, instead

A Leap of Faith

of being stuck once per incident (whether it be to draw blood for lab work or to start an IV lead), it would take two, three, sometimes four sticks to get in a good vein. As you can imagine, after eight months of this I needed a break.

I started the strict diet regimen immediately. I highly recommend the diet to anyone. When I began this diet, I was about three to four weeks out from my last chemotherapy treatment. As anyone who has been through chemotherapy will tell you, it makes you feel miserable. There are all kinds of undesirable side effects. One of them is that your energy level is diminished. After a day, maybe a day and a half of being on this diet I was amazed at how my overall energy and well-being improved. It was like night and day. I would not have thought I could feel that much different over the course of less than two days. The diet is essentially a back to basics diet. Fresh, uncooked fruits and vegetables, whole grains, nuts and seeds. No sugar, absolutely no sugar. No processed food, period. No white flour, none. See a pattern? Only raw fruits and vegetables, whole grains and nuts and seeds, no processed foods of any kind. I felt great, with one exception: I had chest congestion (from the cancer), which caused me to cough constantly, which gave me a sore throat. While the chemotherapy could not cure the cancer, it did (along with the accompanying steroids), keep the inflammation in my lungs to a minimum. Once I was no longer receiving chemotherapy, my lungs became more congested. However, it did not get progressively worse. It is my belief that the pure diet, while insufficient to cure the cancer, was able to hold it at bay. (That is not a medical opinion, just my own personal belief, based on my personal experience). This went on for about 3 months. I did not get any worse, and I felt great with regards to energy level, however, my throat ached all the time. After three months, I was tired of having a sore throat all the time. I was tired of my throat hurting every time I ate. Therefore, I decided I was ready for needles again. I was ready to start the treatment.

In early June of 2001, I started on the vitamins and enzymes (the treatment recommends starting these vitamins and enzymes a couple of weeks before the intravenous treatment, to get these nutrients to the necessary level in my body). A couple of weeks later, I began taking the intravenous treatments. Within a couple of *weeks*, my congestion went away, my coughing stopped, and my sore throat disappeared. The standard regimen calls for intravenous treatments every other day (three times a week), for three weeks, then reduced to once a week for several weeks. After three weeks, once I started on one intravenous treatment per week, my congestion returned. The doctor told me to resume three treatments a week, which I did, and the congestion disappeared again. I am happy to say that nine years later I am Alive and Well. With all due respect to the doctors in Jacksonville who treated me with chemotherapy, God had the final say.

(I am not claiming that this treatment cured my cancer. I used this alternative, and I started feeling better, and am alive and well nine years later. I will leave it up to the individual to make his or her own conclusion as to whether it was coincidence or some other explanation.)

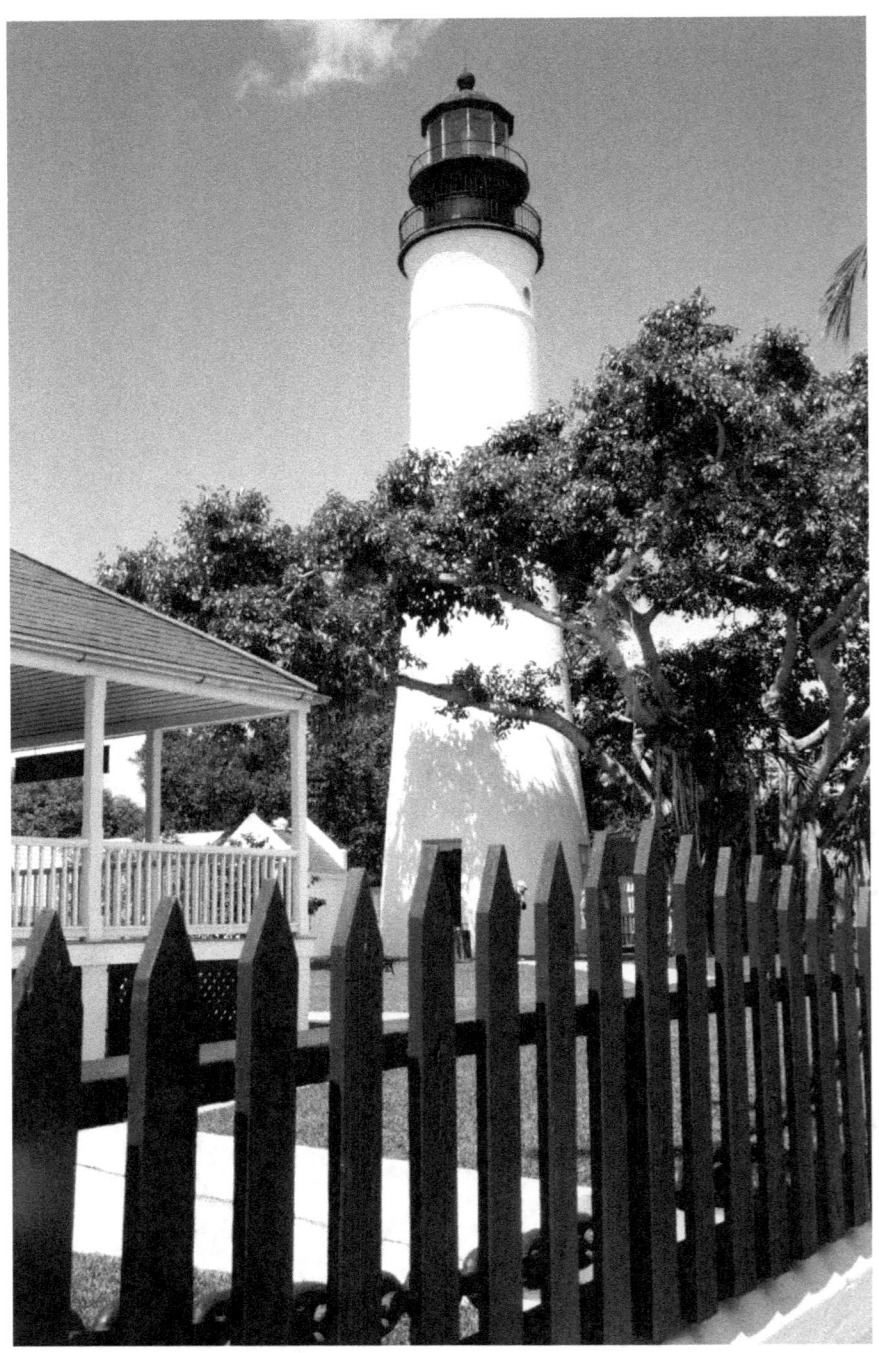

Chapter 12

An All-Encompassing Approach

Successfully battling an illness requires an all-encompassing approach. If you only attack the disease medically, your chances of success are limited. There are many factors involved in dealing with an illness. The medical treatment is just one facet of many. Nutrition is a very important one, but often overlooked. You will have to educate yourself with regards to nutrition, but you should consult a nutritionist and as always consult your doctor before making changes in your diet. The spiritual component is important as well, to include a positive attitude, inner peace, dealing with unforgiveness, realizing that it is not all on your shoulders. Getting plenty of rest is important. Though it may seem cliché and trite, a positive attitude is important. If you can concentrate on all these things (as well as others I am certainly leaving out), your chances of getting better are dramatically improved. This is not a medical opinion or proven fact (other than by my personal experience, probably not an adequate sample to constitute a formal study); it is just a personal opinion that I am sure is shared by many.

As I have already recounted, my faith was an integral part of my healing. Through family members, friends, former churches, there were people all across this country praying for my when I was sick. There were even people across the world praying for me. At the time I got sick, I was participating in an internet community of fans of the professional football team, the Cincinnati Bengals. (Insert your joke here about whether the Bengals are professionals, and whether there are any fans outside of Cincinnati, much less foreign countries, etc.) There were people in this group in England, Italy, and Australia, among other places. While we mostly communicated about football, personal topics would sometimes enter the discussion. I shared some basic information about what I was going through. I did not think about the impact of that community, until one of the members pointed out, "You know, because of this discussion board, you have people all over the world praying for you". Even now, the caring and generosity demonstrated by virtual strangers (no pun intended) humbles me.

The company of friends and loved ones can be very helpful in fighting a disease such as cancer. If you spend a lot of time alone, you dwell on your illness and tend to worry more and get depressed (going back to the importance of a positive attitude). If you do what you can to stay busy, and spend time with friends and family, you are more likely to keep a positive attitude, which can go a long way to helping your recovery. I know they say laughter is the best medicine, but just having someone there to spend time with you is very encouraging and helpful as well; if you can laugh together, all the better. Rent a funny movie and watch it with a friend, play board games, or maybe just reminisce about the good old days. Too often, people do not want to be around the sick person, or they do not want to intrude, but take it from someone who has been there, a visit from a friend or loved one is good medicine. So for those of you, who know someone who is going through this, spend some time with him or her. Do not overestimate a visit from yourself. Just knowing a friend cares enough to pick up and travel across the country, or even across town, can go a long way. Jim, an old Air Force buddy of mine, flew in from San Antonio, Texas to visit. The couple that we met in Key West a few months before I got sick traveled down from Ohio to see me. Another friend from Georgia drove down to see me. Rick, my old Air Force buddy that lived in Jacksonville, visited me regularly. I felt like George Bailey in "It's a Wonderful Life". For those of you who have never seen the greatest Christmas movie ever made, there is a quote in that movie that goes, "Remember George, no man is a failure who has friends." One of my nurses gave me a book about fishing, "Flyfishing for Redfish." It was either her father's or he recommended the book. Even though I like to fish, I never did read the book. Though we have moved many times in the ensuing years, I have held on to that book. It reminds me of my experience, and the generosity of people who did not even know me. I plan to read it one of these days.

A getaway can really help ease the strain of a major illness. The daily routine, the familiar setting of your home and community, can start to close in on the sick person. Depending on the individual situation, going to work, going out to eat or a movie may be strictly limited or prohibited due to the possibility of infection. If at all possible, take a vacation or a short getaway to a secluded spot. A family from our church had a cabin in North Carolina near Lake Lure, and they graciously suggested that we use their cabin for a few days (in January of 2001). This provided us with a wonderful respite from all the stress and turmoil of my ordeal. We had fires in the fireplace, ate out a local restaurant, and drove up to the Blue Ridge Parkway near Asheville, NC and played in the snow with our (almost) two year-old son. It was great to get away to the mountains and just relax. There is no way to quantify how helpful that trip was to my state of mind.

For the first few months of my treatments, I was feeling reasonably well, but because of the nature of my work (sheetrock dust, fumes, mold, etc.) and the location of my cancer (lungs) I could not work. I had a lot of time on my hands. I watched a lot of TV. One of the channels I watched most was the Food Network. I had always liked to cook, but my repertoire was very limited (Hamburger Helper, Tuna Helper, and baked chicken with green peppers drizzled with honey.) That was about all I could make. I watched Emeril Lagasse, Bobby Flay, and Good Eats with Alton Brown. In addition to vastly improving my food knowledge, these shows gave me something to lift my spirits and take my attention off my illness. When I was not feeling weak from the chemotherapy, I was even able to practice some of what I saw and developed my cooking skills.

Something else that can get overlooked is the little stuff. While our needs were met (bills paid, food provided), there is still the day-to-day things that need to be done. A good friend of ours from church, Brad, had his own lawn care business. While I was sick, he took care of our lawn for free. We did not ask him to do this, he just offered. You could volunteer to clean the house or do the laundry. You can go to the grocery and fill up a cart of groceries and take it to them (or cook a meal for them). You can offer to watch the kids for them. Do not wait for people to ask for help, because most people will not ask. Ask God to show you what they need and do it. You can volunteer yourself to transport people to doctor's appointments. Daniel turned one year old just a few months before I got sick. Taking care of a one-year-old and a husband with cancer can be overwhelming. Several of our friends had young children also, and they would take Daniel for the day for a play date; this gave Linda the opportunity to spend some time alone, a much-needed respite. Additionally, during pickup and drop-off, Linda got to spend quality time with the other mom. I am sure Linda got tired of having only a sick husband and a one-year-old to talk to all the time. All the little things help, as a family that is dealing with cancer can get exhausted from the emotional strain, not just the physical things. It is amazing how mental and emotional stress can run you down physically.

Nutrition is one aspect that was sorely lacking in my treatment plan. Hippocrates, the ancient Greek physician, who is considered the Western "Father of Medicine", said, "Let food be thy medicine, and let medicine be thy food." Hippocrates held the belief that the body must be treated as a whole, not just a series of parts. He believed in the natural healing process of rest, a good diet, fresh air and cleanliness. Invariably, some will contend that these are old-fashioned ideas that are irrelevant in light of modern advances in medicine. But perhaps we have abandoned good principles and blindly latched on to medicine, believing that only medicine can save us, instead of using medicine to augment good fundamental principles of health. Increasing numbers of people are turning to food and nutrition as a weapon in their arsenal for good health. According to Plunkett Research, in 2009, "The hottest growth areas in the food business are in natural foods, organic products, health foods, diet foods, and nutritionally-enhanced foods." (Footnote_4)

Chemotherapy attacks all of your body, not just cancer cells. It degrades your immune system. If I had known then what I know now, I would have consumed foods that boost the immune system, and avoided foods (like sugar and processed foods) that compromise the immune system. I do not know if this aspect of cancer treatment has changed since I went through it, but in my opinion, it would be a good idea for anyone who is dealing with cancer to seek out a nutritionist for information on this subject. Most doctors have neither the time nor the training to focus on your nutrition, so you have to be self-educated and proactive.

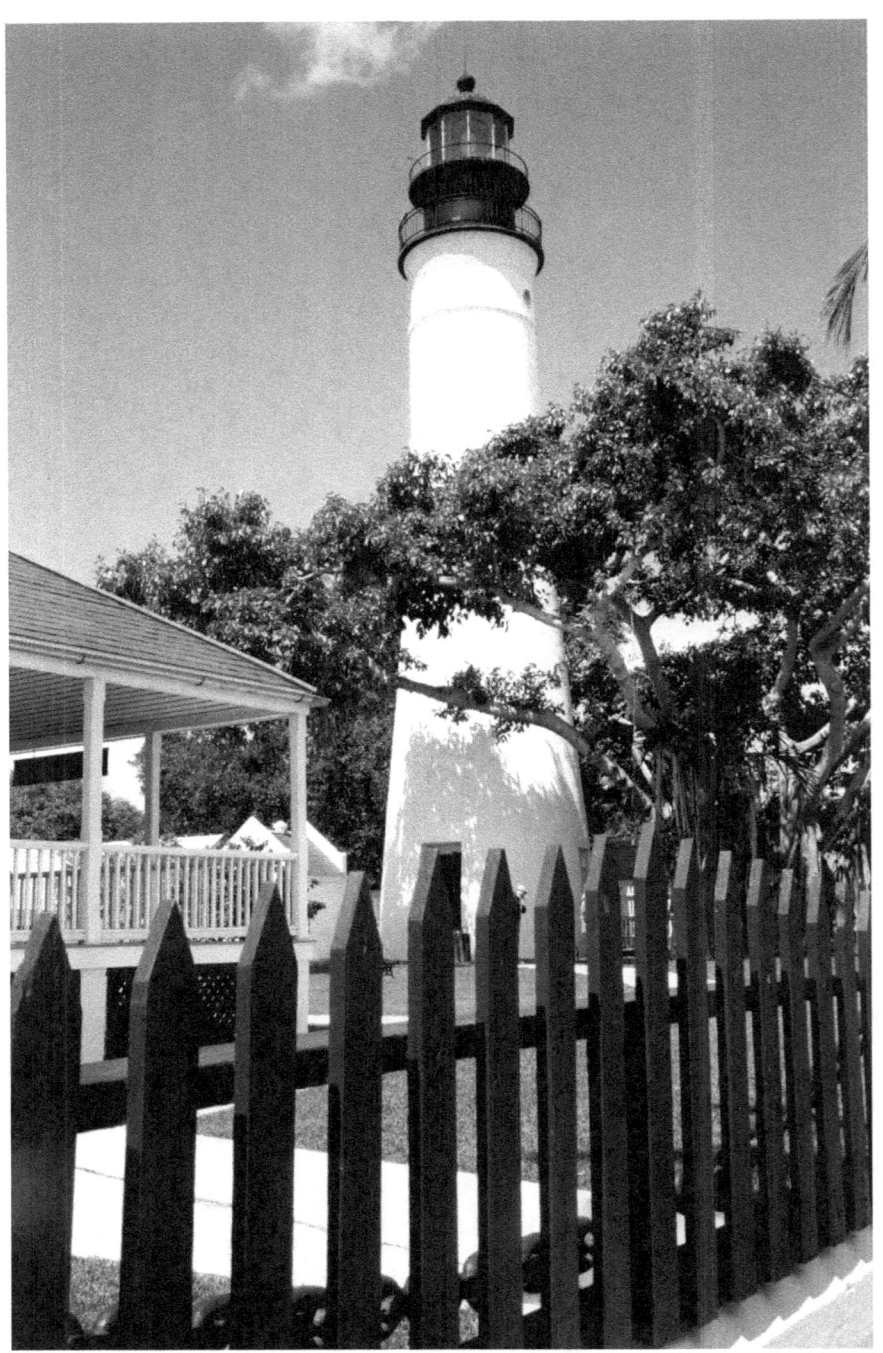

Chapter 13

Perfect Love Casts Out Fear

One of the most significant ways in which cancer attacks is through fear. When most people find out they have cancer, the first emotion they experience is fear. This fear can range from a mild fear to one that is overwhelming. As I said in an earlier chapter, I believe cancer is the most feared word in the English language.

What are the effects of fear? Physical effects of anxiety (or fear) may include: heart palpitations, muscle weakness and tension, fatigue, nausea, chest pain, shortness of breath, stomach aches or headaches. While these may be extreme effects of anxiety, even milder instances of these effects would have a negative impact on a person's ability to fight off a disease.

2 Timothy 1:7

For God has not given us a spirit of fear, but of power and of love and of a sound mind.

This scripture contrasts a spirit of fear with a spirit of power, love, and a sound mind. The logical conclusion is that we either have the spirit of fear OR the spirit of power, love, and a sound mind. While there is no way to quantify the effects of either on a person's health or recovery from disease, common sense and intelligence dictate that the spirit of power, love, and a sound mind will have a more positive and helpful effect than a spirit of fear.

Matthew 10:28

And do not fear those who kill the body but cannot kill the soul. But rather fear Him who is able to destroy both soul and body in hell.

One thing that can affect the level of stress and anxiety that a person has is their inner peace. For me, inner peace is knowing that I have peace with God through my Lord and Savior Jesus Christ. This is true in everyday living, but is magnified greatly in

Perfect Love Casts Out Fear

the face of a potentially terminal disease. If a person is facing the
possibility of death from disease, and is uncertain what eternity
holds for him, that uncertainty can produce tremendous stress. On
the other hand, if a person is at peace with their eternal destiny,
the possibility of dying from a disease holds little stress, other
than the stress of leaving behind loved ones (spouse, children,
etc.). This difference, while not the deciding factor in survival
from an illness, can make a big difference in a person's recovery.

We all have things we fear, but if we have placed our trust in
Jesus, if we are Christians, then we should not fear death. I am not
saying we should desire death or tempt fate, but if we truly
believe the Bible, then we should not fear death. The gospel is all
about: realizing we are a sinner, deserving of death and hell after
we die; Jesus coming to earth, sharing our humanity and living a
perfect life in our place; Jesus dying on the cross for our sins; God
raising Jesus from death to eternal life, that we who trust in Him
should follow after Him and share in eternal life in heaven.

Romans 8:15

For you did not receive a spirit that makes you a slave again to fear, but
you received the Spirit of sonship. And by him we cry, "Abba, Father."

As I alluded to in an earlier chapter, when I found out I had
cancer, I had no fear. God brought to my remembrance that I had
eternal life through His Son Jesus, therefore even if the cancer
were unto death, I had no reason to fear; I would be with Him in
paradise.

God Said Net Yet!

As you have probably noticed, there is a recurring theme here with regards to fear. The key to overcoming fear is faith in God through His Son Jesus. I am not saying that if you are trusting in God, you will never be afraid of spiders or snakes or clowns. However, when it comes to dealing with death or debilitating fears, I believe that a true faith in God through His Son Jesus will free you from fear.

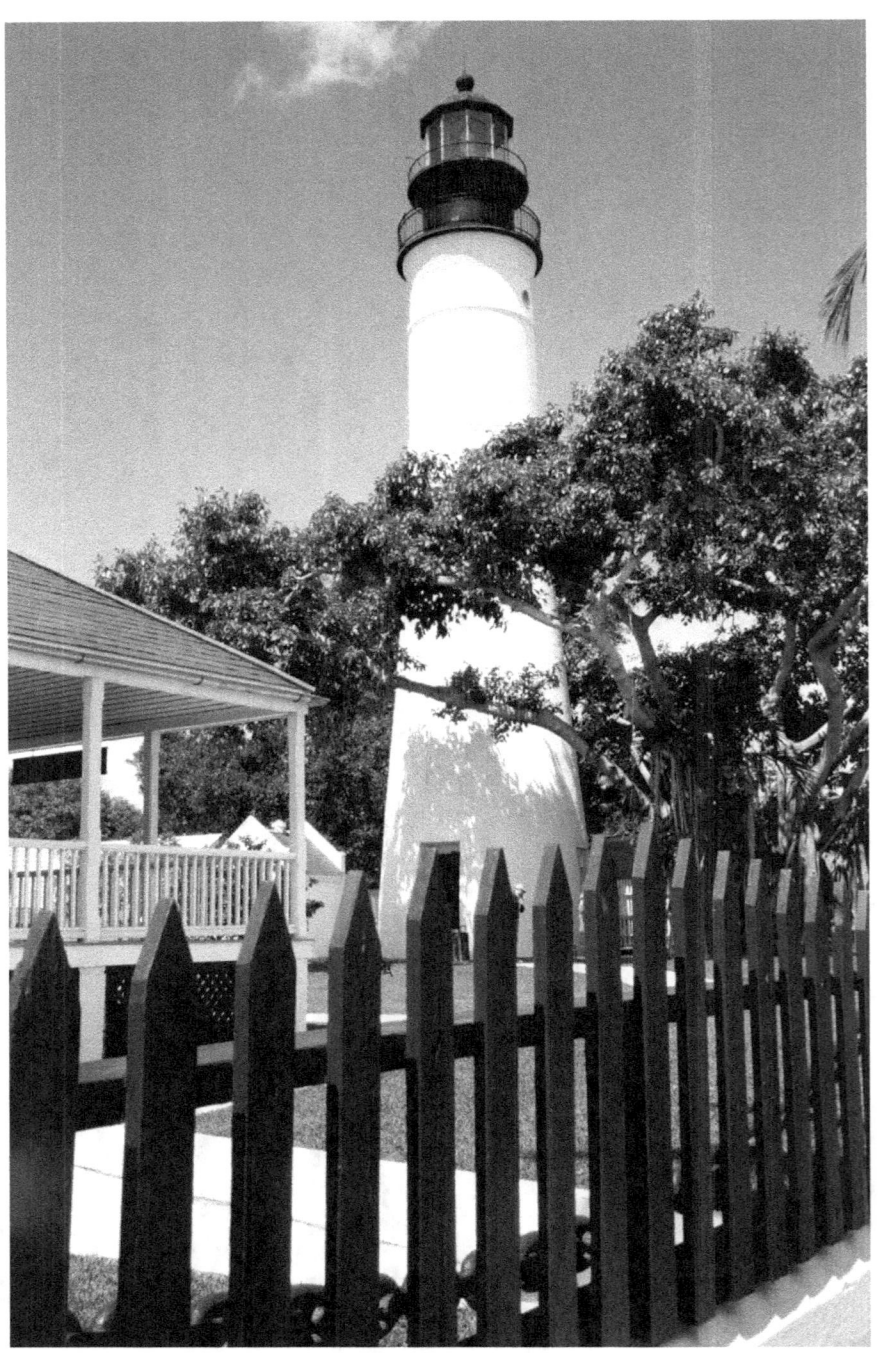

Chapter 14

A Foolproof Diet I Discovered on the Way To Recovering from "Terminal Cancer"

(A disclaimer I would like to make up front is that this diet is something that worked for me and is derived from my own experience and opinion. I am not, nor do I claim to be, a nutritional expert. All claims and statements about this diet are simply my observations on what worked for me personally. Everyone should consult a qualified nutritionist or dietician, and his or her doctor, before starting any diet or nutritional regimen.)

119

God Said Net Yet!

Diets are really very simple, what complicates the issue is the fact that people want some magic formula or pill that will allow them to eat anything they want and still lose (or maintain) weight. The truth is that there are certain foods and ingredients that cause weight gain and these foods and ingredients must be limited to very small portions (or eliminated altogether) in order to lose (or maintain) weight. You have to be willing to make choices (sacrifices) in respect to food, but most people are not willing to. People want to be able to eat ice cream and french fries and drink sodas and still lose (or maintain) weight.; unless you are burning a gazillion calories a day, this is not possible.

After walking away from conventional medical treatment for cancer, I followed an alternative treatment that included a strict diet designed to help the body's natural ability to fight cancer. Through this diet, I realized that the same things which can make us more susceptible to cancer can also cause us to gain/retain unwanted weight: sugar, white flour, processed food, preservatives and additives. It seems very self-evident, but a basic whole food diet will not only make you feel better (and arguably stay healthier), but also help you to stay trim. Staying trim will in turn give you more energy and make you feel better (there is a kind of multiplication effect). Within a couple of days of beginning this diet, I was amazed at how much energy I had. (In addition, I was just three to four weeks past my final chemotherapy treatment.) I did not have to nap during the day, I felt great and my energy level was high; a stark contrast to a few days before when I was still eating the old way (sugar, processed food, few vegetables). Again, this is not a scientific study, just personal experience, but I saw within days (not weeks or months) the effects of a good diet.

A Foolproof Diet

I could not deny the benefits of a diet that could make me (someone still dealing with the side effects of chemotherapy) feel so dramatically different, almost instantly (less than two full days after starting the diet). I was sold on the first part of this alternative plan immediately.

After reading Dr. Binzel's book, although I was open to the alternative treatment, I needed a break from needles so I was not ready to start the treatment. I did, however, begin following the diet immediately and assiduously. Within a few weeks, I was able to fit in size 34 pants. I had not worn that size since my teen years.

Raw fruits and vegetables, that is the starting point, all fresh and uncooked, and more vegetables than fruits (maybe 70/30, or 60/40, you have to find a balance that feels right to you). Why fresh? You want the maximum nutritional value from the food. If it has been canned, it is not as nutritional as fresh. If is has been frozen, it is a good bet that the fruit/vegetable was blanched (or cooked partially) to preserve color and texture. Why raw? There are enzymes in fresh fruits and vegetables, which are destroyed or deactivated when the food is heated above a certain temperature. Although your body is able to synthesize these enzymes from other sources, if your body is required to perform this task, resources are being taxed that could be used for other things. By eating all your fruits and vegetables raw, you get the enzymes straight into your body. This is especially important when you are fighting a disease like cancer. However, if you are undergoing traditional treatment like chemotherapy, it is very important to consult your doctor with regards to your diet, because chemotherapy diminishes your immune system, making you dangerously susceptible to bacteria that might be found in raw fruits and vegetables.

Only whole grains are permitted on this diet (whole wheat, brown rice, etc.). While grains that have been processed are fortified with the established (by government) necessary nutrients, it is always best to get nutrients in their naturally occurring form, rather than a fortified food or a supplement. Also, can we really be certain that we know everything that is in whole grain wheat or brown rice, which is essential to good health?

Nuts, seeds, and berries. Of course, as fresh as possible, and avoid frozen or dried berries if at all possible. The nutritional content of nuts, seeds, and berries is immense and as varied as the foods themselves. As with all foods, be careful of processed foods (for example, honey-roasted nuts, which are high in sugar, or cereals with dried berries or fruit).

The old food pyramid is a good starting point for a healthy diet, however there are some flaws. Bread, cereal, rice and pastas make up the lower tier, and the group of food that should be consumed most. This can be detrimental if the cereals and grains you are consuming are not whole grain. Most breads contain in large part (if not 100%) processed wheat that has been stripped of its nutrition and then fortified. Also, most if not all store-bought bread contains sugar, corn syrup, preservatives and additives. Cereal: I challenge you to find, on an average grocery store shelf, a cereal that does not contain significant amounts of processed flour and sugar and preservatives: even the ones that seem to be "healthy." Rice, the vast majority of rice that is consumed is white rice, which has been processed, and is nutritionally deficient like white flour. The same goes for pasta. Not only will large portions of processed grains compromise your health, but these will also cause weight gain.

The food pyramid lists sweets and oils at the top, recommending that these items be consumed sparingly. This is good advice, especially with regards to sweets, however, when it comes to cooking oils, you need to do your homework: all oils are not created equally. Olive oil, extra virgin olive oil, is perhaps the healthiest oil (there have been studies that suggest olive oil raises your good cholesterol and lowers your bad cholesterol. This claim is not made about any other cooking oil.)

What is not to be consumed on this diet is almost as important as what is to be consumed. Number one would be sugar. Voluminous material has been published on the unhealthy effects of sugar. However, I would caution against substituting alternative sweeteners, as most of these can be harmful as well. Personally I use honey as a substitute (I use honey to sweeten my coffee.) Next would be white flour (flour that has had all the nutrients processed, bleached white, and then fortified with nutrients). Again, there is a significant amount of information out there regarding the ill effects of white flour. The third big no-no is processed foods. Processed foods are detrimental for numerous reasons: undesired weight gain; a weakened immune system; and toxins which make the body work harder to eliminate. Processed foods cause weight gain, because they are loaded with low-nutrient, high-calorie ingredients like white flour and sugar. Weight gain has been shown in some studies (and referenced by the American Cancer Society) to increase the risk of cancer. In addition, white flour and sugar have been shown to be detrimental to the immune system. Our immune system helps protect us from and fight against diseases like cancer. Finally, all the preservatives and additives in processed foods are toxins, which require extra work by our body to process and dispose of. While it is nearly impossible to avoid processed foods completely, the less you consume the better.

I concede that avoiding processed food completely is very difficult. Processed foods are everywhere, and with our busy lives, it is not always practical to prepare and eat whole foods. The key is keeping processed food to an absolute minimum.

Meat should be limited. For one thing, the more meat you eat the less fruits, vegetables and grains you are likely to eat. You need protein, but it should be a limited percentage of your overall intake. I personally am not an opponent of red meat, nor a proponent of poultry. Again, this is my personal opinion, not professional dietary advice. I think all meats are good in moderation. Given the amount of antibiotics and hormones that some poultry contains, the negatives may outweigh the benefit of lower cholesterol. Fish is one of the healthiest protein sources you can consume, but we must consider the "processed" factor even with fish. "Processed fish?!" you say. Yes, most fish you will find at your local supermarket are farm raised, not wild. Farm raised salmon, for example, do not feed on the same diet as wild salmon, but they are given man made feed. Some farm raised salmon is reported to have toxins in them due to the feed they are given. Also, farm raised salmon normally have a very unappealing gray color to the flesh. Therefore, either farm-raised salmon are given feed which has additives that turn the flesh pink, or they are injected with a dye to give the flesh that characteristic pink color. With regards to poultry, if you can find and afford them, farm-raised, cage free, hormone/antibiotic free protein sources are best.

A Foolproof Diet

Regardless of what kind of protein sources you are consuming, keeping the percentage of meat (in relation to your overall diet) you consume low is most important. Those who believe that B17 can fight cancer stress that your natural defense system uses certain enzymes, the same ones that your body uses to digest animal protein, to fight cancer. (footnote_5)

Sticking to this diet religiously can be very difficult. The reality is that it is very difficult to take the time and effort to eat right. Everyone's life is so hectic, that it is often times much easier to wolf down some fast food or a frozen dinner than to make a meal from scratch with fresh ingredients. I was able to do it because I was faced with terminal cancer: my life depended on success. However, since getting better, I admit there have been times when I have fallen off the wagon and gotten back on sodas and candy and processed foods. One of the benefits of sharing my story through this book is that it has renewed my commitment to eating a pure diet. At the time of this writing, I am almost as zealous with my diet as I was when I was recovering from cancer. While it took grit and determination to get back on this regimen, it has now become habit, and the feeling of well-being is so worth it. While it is not vital (for someone who is following this diet for weight-loss or general health) to be as assiduous in adherence to this diet, just keep in mind that every time you consume sugar or white flour or processed food, you are degrading your health and very likely gaining weight (in my opinion).

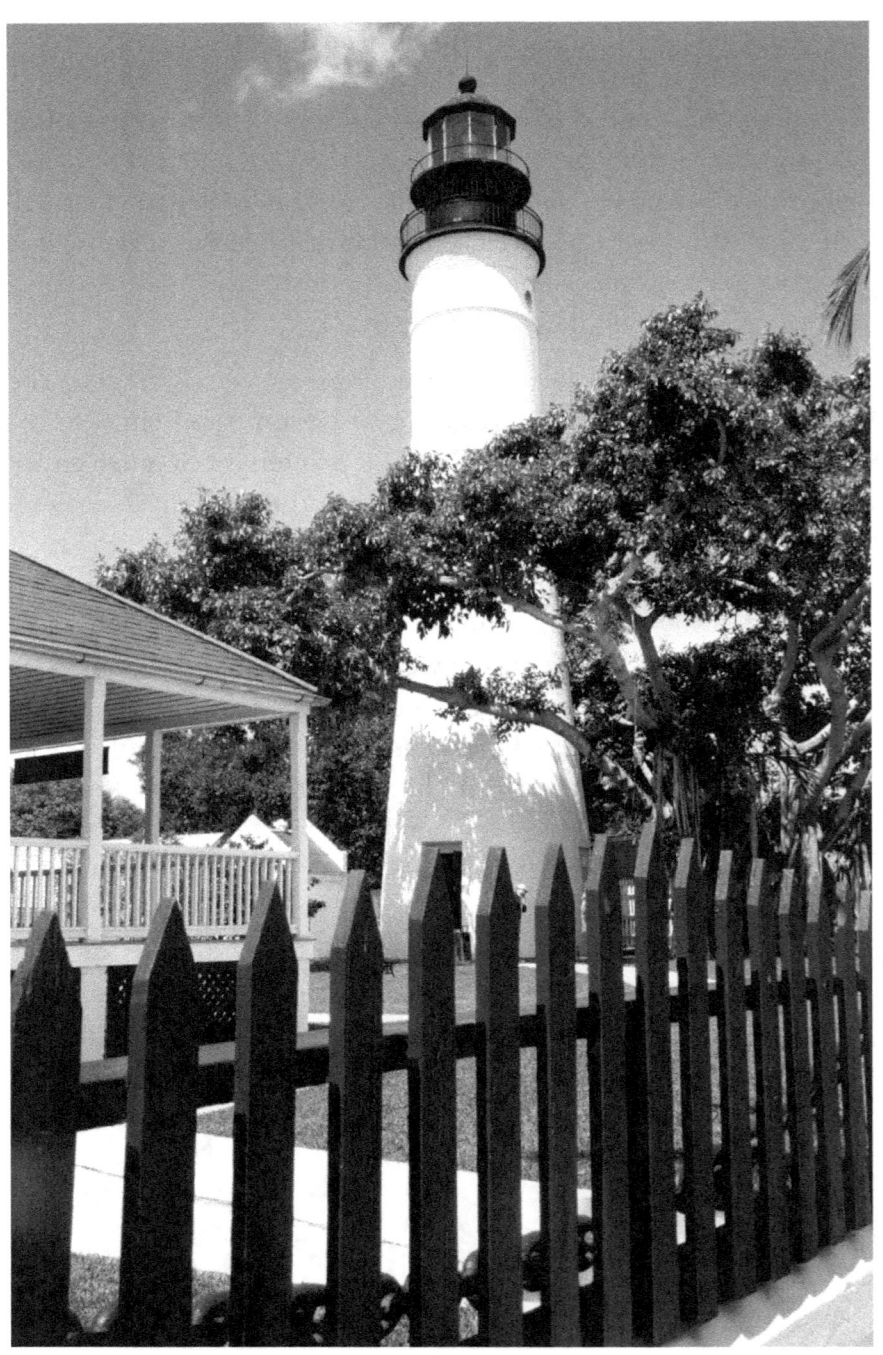

Chapter 15

A Place for Kids

As soon as I started feeling better, I knew that I was supposed to step out and get back into the business of working with teenagers. I was not clear on exactly how that was to play out, but I knew that I was supposed to return to my calling to work with troubled youth. I had always disagreed with a lot of the methods used in group home models, and wanted to start and run my own place for kids. I wanted to implement all the techniques and ideas that I thought worked, and replace the ineffective techniques with ideas of my own. Either I was idealistic or naïve, but I believed I could raise support and open a home for kids.

Heat and humidity does not sit well with me personally. As a matter of fact, hot and humid climates make me feel miserable. This kind of weather saps all my energy and makes me feel sick. I have always noticed this, but after getting cancer, and the search I went through trying to ascertain what might have caused it, I came to the conclusion that the weather in Florida was one of the factors that contributed to my getting cancer. I read an article a few years after recovering from cancer, which cited that Jacksonville, FL was one of the top five cities in the U.S. for lung cancer deaths. (In 2009, according to the American Cancer Society, only California had more deaths from lung cancer than Florida.) While that statistic is likely attributable, in part, to the large proportion of retired people in the state of Florida, I believe the weather (as well as other environmental conditions) is also a factor. Therefore, staying in Florida to pursue the goal of opening a home for kids was not an option to me; I was determined to move north, to a milder climate. I longed to move back to the Greater Cincinnati area, where I had grown up, but I did not have any contacts other than some cousins that I had not kept in touch with for years. Taryl and Marcia, our new friends, whom we had met in Key West just months before I got sick, lived in Mentor, OH (near Cleveland, OH) and had many contacts whom we thought could be helpful in our endeavor. Before I had even started the alternative treatment for my cancer, before I had even started to recover, we made a trip to Mentor, OH to visit our friends and begin networking for contacts. I was stepping out in faith, because I knew that God was in the process of healing me and He was calling me to do this. I took my Southern Belle out of the South and moved her to 'Ninevah'. Daniel was only two years old and loved to travel. We found a place in Ashtabula, a quaint little city on Lake Erie at the mouth of the Ashtabula River. An interesting note, the word Ashtabula comes from an Algonquin Indian term meaning "river of many fish." I did some fishing while we lived there, and I did not catch "many fish", so either I am an incompetent fisherman or things have changed in the last few hundred years since the river was named by the Indians.

After nearly a year in Ashtabula, it became clear to me that opening a home for kids in Ohio was more my idea than God's idea. Linda was unable to find full-time work, and I was met with closed doors everywhere I turned. We were having trouble paying basic bills, and there seemed to be no prospects. After much praying and seeking with Linda, I discerned that I needed to give up, for now, the dream of having our own place for kids and seek employment at an established group home. Although working with kids in Ohio was not to be, I believe that our time there was an important part of the healing process for me from cancer. Experiencing the seasons changing on the banks of Lake Erie, exploring new health food options, and being involved in fishing and photography helped heal my whole body, strengthening me for the time ahead when we would pour our lives into the lives of hurting youth.

We began a search for group homes that hired couples to live with kids in a group home setting. We applied to four group homes: one in Ohio; two in Texas; and one in Maine. "Now hold on!" you might be saying, "I thought you left Florida to get away from hot, humid climates. You hypocrite!" While it gets very hot in Texas, some parts of Texas are very dry, and it is the *humid* heat that really gets to me. I spent six weeks in San Antonio for basic training, I lived in Southwest Oklahoma, and I traveled extensively throughout Texas, so I was very familiar with the weather in Texas. Other than the Gulf Coast, most of Texas is relatively dry. One of the group homes we looked at was in San Antonio, and the other was in Amarillo. A vivid memory I have from my Air Force days brings home the difference between "dry heat" and "humid heat." I played a lot of intramural softball while I was in the Air Force. Since I was a pretty good ball player, I was given time off my shifts in the control tower to represent our squadron on the field. One June day, we played a game from 5:00 PM to 6:00 PM. While it was definitely hot, it did not seem oppressively hot to me. I finished the game and returned to the control tower to complete my shift. Weather being an integral part of aviation, each base had its own weather reporting station, and we received frequent weather updates in the tower in order that we could inform the pilots and stay abreast of changing weather ourselves. When I got backed to the tower and checked the most recent weather report, I was amazed to see the temperature: 113 degrees! 113 degrees at 6:00 PM! I would never have guessed the temperature was that high, but it didn't seem that hot because there was very little humidity. Some people make jokes and think there is little difference, "when it's hot - it's hot, regardless of the humidity." Maybe others don't notice the difference, but I know I do. I would rather have that dry 113 degree heat than 90 degrees (with humidity to match) any day.

We visited the group home in Ohio and interviewed in person, but just submitted resumes via mail, and interviewed over the phone with the other group homes. While we were waiting to hear back from the group homes we had applied to, the group

A Place for Kids

home in Maine called us and offered us a job. After prayer and consideration, we believed strongly that it was the right fit for us, so we accepted. There was just one problem; we lacked the funds to move from Ohio to Maine. But we knew that God was leading us in that direction, so we went to Him, requesting assistance with our need. Out of the blue, completely unexpected (or more accurately, in answer to our prayer), we received a check for $7,000. We were humbled and amazed. Not only did we have enough money to move to Maine, but we were able to pay for one of those companies that loads the moving van, drives it to your destination, and unloads everything for you. All we had to do was pack and unpack our boxes. This enabled us to take our time, see Niagara Falls on the way, and drive up the coast of Southern Maine. If you've never been to Maine, it is even more scenic and beautiful than you've imagined.

We spent four years in Maine, and thoroughly enjoyed our time there. We visited just about every corner of the state, including a good part of New Hampshire and Massachusetts. We took a vacation to Cape Cod one summer that was one of those truly memorable vacations. Cape Cod was every bit as picturesque and charming as I had envisioned. Statuesque lighthouses, inviting beaches, sandy cliffs, quaint little towns, and seafood, oh the seafood! From our jumping off point in Hyannis, we visited sights from Provincetown at the tip of the Cape, to Martha's Vineyard, covering almost every square mile of Cape Cod (okay, maybe a *slight* exaggeration). We took the ferry to the Martha's Vineyard, planning to use public transportation to see the sights while we spent the day on the island. While walking around Oak Bluffs, the harbor town where you disembark from the ferry, we saw a business that rented out basic Jeep Wranglers for exploring the island. Fully expecting the price to be prohibitive (like several hundred dollars for the day), I decided to check it out anyway. I was shocked and elated to find out that the Jeeps rented for just $99 for the whole day! We got a yellow Jeep and explored the whole island on our terms and our schedule. If I had to pick one attraction on Martha's Vineyard that I would recommend, it would be Gay Head Cliffs. Located on the Southwest corner of the island, the cliffs are truly a spectacular sight; the different colors of sand and clay, contrasting with the green grass, blue skies, white clouds, and blue-green water must be seen to be truly appreciated. We were treated to a beautiful day, some beautiful sights, and some delicious seafood on Martha's Vineyard. To top it all off, a gorgeous sunset was the backdrop for a smooth ferry ride across the Atlantic Ocean back to the mainland.

One of activities we enjoyed most of all in Maine was moose-hunting. Not the kind with guns (not that there's anything wrong with that), but driving around trying to spot moose. Although they are somewhat like cows with long legs, moose are really spectacular to see in the wild, especially the males with their magnificent antlers. Moose, for the most part, are gentle and non-aggressive. However, you want to avoid males when they are in the rut during mating season and mother moose with their young. Mother moose protecting their young are reportedly some of the most dangerous animals in North America. Also, great care is required when driving at night in Maine, due to the nature of moose-car collisions. Because of the moose' long legs and extremely heavy trunks, a large number of people are killed when running into moose. The bulk of a moose's body is above the level of the hood of most cars. When a car hits a moose head-on, the legs get chopped, and the body of the moose falls through the windshield, crushing the driver. Moose move slowly and since they fear no predator, tend not to look at oncoming vehicles (which would reflect the headlights showing they are there), and their dark coat blends into the dark background of the night. But if you are careful, and persistent, you are likely to be treated to seeing many moose while traveling around the state of Maine.

Although driving around looking for moose, or sitting at one of the salt dumps waiting for them to amble up from the woods, was very enjoyable, those experiences paled in comparison to a couple of encounters I had in the wild. On one occasion, I was hiking in Baxter State Park (home of Mount Katahdin, the northern terminus of the Appalachian Trail), taking pictures of the serene landscape: pristine wilderness lakes with mountains in the background. I was standing on a foot bridge that spanned a section of one of the lakes, when I saw a large bull moose come out of the woods and enter the water to cross the lake, about 30 yards away from me. I sat down on the bridge to steady my camera and take some pictures of this magnificent moose. When he heard me, he stopped in his tracks, and slowly turned his head to look at me. He just stood there staring at me for a few seconds. Although I know moose are normally gentle creatures, it was still a little scary to have this 1,000 pound wild beast standing there staring at me. An average adult male moose stands 6-7 feet high at the shoulders (not the head) and weighs 850-1500 pounds! I remained very still, and he turned his head back and went on his way.

Another encounter took place in the Allagash Wilderness Waterway, where you are almost guaranteed to see moose. The Allagash Wilderness Waterway is a 92 mile corridor of connected lakes, rivers and streams in Northwest Maine. There is no development, aside from basic Forest Ranger stations, and no electricity in the entire waterway. It is a place where you can really "get away from it all." A remote wilderness refuge, the Allagash takes several hours to reach on gravel roads, dodging logging trucks, from the nearest town. Every summer, several trips were organized to take some of the kids from the group home on week-long canoe and camping trips in the Allagash. We loaded up in a 15 passenger van, hauling a trailer with the canoes and gear, and made the long trip to the northern put-in point. All the camping gear, a dozen campers (including the chaperones), and food for a week were loaded into the various canoes and we set off across the windswept lake. Paddling across the lakes, against the wind, in a canoe weighed down with supplies to one of the primitive camping sites was an arduous task, but there was a real sense of accomplishment and a job well done when we reached our destination. (Well that is what I told the boys to keep them going.) After unloading and setting up camp, the boys enjoyed fishing and swimming while we (I) prepared a gourmet camp dinner. I made a pseudo Alfredo sauce from pancake batter, butter, milk and cream cheese. Mark, one of our chaperones and a registered Maine guide, was beside himself over the meal. He kept repeating "Are you kidding me right now?" Mark was thoroughly impressed with my cooking skills; so much so that he said that he was either going to make me his cook, when he started his full-time guiding service, or he was going to marry me. I told him that he would have to settle for making me his cook since I was already spoken for. After a delicious, filling meal we settled in for the evening around a crackling campfire. As night approached, we lay on the gravel beach of the lake, watching commercial jets streaking high across the twilight sky, and listening to the cry of the loon (and sometimes coyotes): a little slice of heaven.

We saw lots of moose in the Allagash, though generally from a great distance. It was difficult to get close to the moose, especially in the middle of the day on an open lake. Mark, knowing that I was an avid amateur photographer who wanted to get some good moose pictures, promised to guide me to a spot where I was certain to get some good shots. One morning, very early, Mark and I headed out to a cove where moose were known to hang out. As we paddled into the cove, we got very quiet and deliberate, taking care not to spook any of the moose. We saw several moose that morning, relatively close up, including a momma and her calf, but the one that was remarkable was a large bull moose out in the middle of the cove. Moose like to feed on the vegetation underwater, and an adult male will eat up to 50 pounds of vegetation per day. This magnificent beast put his head underwater to feed, then after a few minutes brought his head up out of the water, and as he did the water ran down off his antlers, spraying into a mist, glistening in the morning sun. Quite a remarkable sight!

Believe it or not, we actually found time amid all our travels to work with kids. We spent about half of our four years there in a girls cottage, and the other half in a boys cottage. There were good times, and tough times. Working with troubled teenagers can be one of the most emotionally trying jobs in the world. With some of the kids, you pour your heart and life into them, and all you get back is venom. You hope and pray that somewhere down the road, a seed that you planted will bear fruit and make a difference in their life. With some it does, as we have seen with kids that we keep in touch with. However, the sad, hard-to-accept truth is that for some, it never will. That was very hard for me, because I wanted to believe that I could make a difference with each and every kid. Perhaps that was too idealistic a notion, but I believed it.

The organization we worked for in Maine, because of the fact that most of their funding came from government sources, had fallen into a pattern of administrating to please the state rather than helping the kids. Unfortunately, this approach grew steadily worse over the course of the four years we were there. We saw the writing on the wall, and also because of our desire to move south to be closer to family, we gave notice and left in the summer of 2006. Within a couple of years, the organization closed down all the cottages and discontinued the residential program. The demise of this organization was very disappointing. Either poor decision making (deciding to rely primarily on state funding), or dependence on state funding (necessitated by a lack of private donations) caused the organization to abandon their mission, and make decisions based on the bottom line rather than what was in the best interests of the youth. Sadly, this led to the organization's downfall.

After spending part of the summer traveling, looking for jobs elsewhere, and visiting friends and family, we settled in Georgetown, KY, believing that we were done working in the group home setting. However, after a two year break in Kentucky, living in the middle of beautiful horse country (the Bluegrass Region) we took a job at a group home in Western North Carolina in the fall of 2008, knowing that we were called to continue in this work. I believe that God led us in moving to North Carolina and taking the job, but it was only to be for a season, a short season.

We settled into the group home in Western North Carolina, and fell in love with the area immediately. We poured ourselves into the job, and although we faced some serious challenges (from kids, families, and administration), we muddled through and continued ministering to the kids and their families through the fall of 2009.

Sometimes life throws you a curve ball. Sometimes things do not work out the way you want them to. We have a plan all laid out, a plan that we believe is the best plan for our life, and when things do not go according to that plan, we feel everything has fallen apart and God could not possibly be involved. However, the key, if you are trusting in God as your guide, is to accept that what happens is God's will. Initially, when we took the houseparent job in North Carolina, we thought we would be there for years. We made plans to start looking for a house or land, we got involved in the community, and we started making the staff apartment our own. We thought we would retire in that job. Western North Carolina is beautiful country, and we had finally found the place where we wanted to settle down and prepare for retirement. (Although, according to Linda, it is not Shangrilusia: Andalusia, AL + Shangrila.)

Just before Thanksgiving, after working there for just over a year, we were terminated without notice and on false terms. At first, we were shocked and our pride was hurt. We could not believe what happened and we wanted justice (either through litigation or just telling off the people who terminated us). But as time wore on, I began to see that God was in control and in the end this was for the best. The group home situation had become very stressful for us, and although I had been trying to spend time working on my book, it was difficult to get any work done. Once we were liberated from that situation, I had time and energy aplenty to work on my book. I believe that my story, a story of hope in the face of death and alternatives to standard cancer treatment, is a powerful story that needs to be heard by many people. I was now able to focus on sharing my story through my book and speaking. Additionally, Linda told me that I would never have a better opportunity to finish my book and that I should go ahead and do it.

It is a passion of mine to share my story of hope and faith with those who are going through the agonizing experience of cancer. Unfortunately, because of the widespread occurrence of cancer in our day, this is a story with universal impact and appeal. Everyone has either experienced cancer themselves or knows someone close to them who has experienced cancer. I have shared this story, as often as I have had opportunity, with individuals and small groups, but this book will allow me to share my story with many more people through the power of the written word.

The more time I spent working on my book, I discovered just how much I enjoyed writing. I discovered that this was what I wanted to do now for a living. I was 46 years old at the time we were terminated from the group home. I did not want to pick up and move again to another group home, and I did not want to continue working in group homes many more years (certainly not until I was 65 years old). Residential youth treatment is definitely a job for younger (younger than 50 year olds) couples with more energy. I do not know for certain how successful this book will be and that other books I write will provide income, but I am stepping out in faith, believing that they will. This book is just the first in many projects that I have in the works. Look for more books from me in the near future. I am very passionate about family, education, politics, and nutrition. The core principle that governs my views on all things is my Christian faith. I also have a fiction novel in the works. I do not want to give away too much information, but it is about a lake with a secret.

This story began in the fall of 1990, when I stopped running from God and surrendered total control of my life to Him. Although the direction of my life, since surrendering to God's will, has not always gone according to my plan, things have always turned out well.

Romans 8:28

And we know that all things work together for good
to those who love God,
to those who are the called according to *His* purpose.

Recommended Reading

Following is a list of resources that helped me personally in my fight with cancer. This is not a professional endorsement, just a personal one.

Alive and Well
by Dr. Philip Binzel

The Little Cyanide Cookbook;
Delicious Recipes Rich in Vitamin B17
by June de Spain

Heinerman's Encyclopedia of Fruits and Vegetables
Heinerman's Encyclopedia of Healing Juices
Heinerman's Encyclopedia of Healing Herbs and Spices
by John Heinerman

Getting Started on Getting Well (a companion to her videos)
by Dr. Lorraine Day

Healing
by Francis McNutt
(of Christian Healing Ministries in Jacksonville, FL)

Footnotes

1. Cancer.org

   http://www.cancer.org/docroot/stt/stt_0.asp?from=fast

2. Harvard.edu

   www.health.harvard.edu

3. (rarediseases.about.com & cancer.org)

   Cancer.org

   http://www.cancer.org/docroot/eto/eto_1_3_bone_marrow.asp

   http://rarediseases.about.com/od/rarediseasesb/a/bmt05.htm

4. Plunkett Research

   http://plunkettresearch.com/Industries/FoodBeverageTobacco/tabid/203/Default.aspx

5. Alive and Well by Dr. Philip Binzel

All of these footnotes were accurate at the time of the writing of this book. I cannot be held responsible for the content of the websites referenced or any changes in web addresses.

Notes